Unleash the Power
of your
Vagus Nerve

A Self-Help Guide to Relieve Anxiety, Reduce Stress, Depression and Improve your Health with Step-by-Step Daily Exercises

By

Arnold Scott

CONTENTS

INTRODUCTION

The human body is an enigma. The entire structure of our anatomy can be perplexing, but as time goes on, so too does our vast amount of knowledge. As we learn more, however, we discover more questions that need to be answered.

Within the body, the brain is the most confounding element. The brain is a complex system of cells that all work in their intricate manner.

What we often forget about are the nerves that connect the brain to the rest of the body. These are referred to as cranial nerves, and there are 12 of them in our bodies. The vagus nerve is classified as the tenth nerve, indicated with a Roman numeral X, and it is one of the few nerves that supports both sensory and motor functions within the body.

This long nerve extends to some of our bodies' most important areas. In this book, we will explore the complex anatomy of this organ to give you a general sense of just what might be affected by a disruption in your vagus nerve.

Many factors could contribute to damage to your vagus nerve. Many symptoms of a disrupted nerve are seemingly unrelated to the nervous system, like stomach aches or back pain. Many individuals will go a while without realizing that a simple stimulation of their vagus nerve could have life-altering effects.

The book begins with a very structured breakdown of what the vagus nerve is, what it affects, and the biology of this complex system. The deeper you can grasp the concept of the vagus nerve, the easier it will be for you to understand the symptoms you experience and how they're related to your vagal system.

By Chapter 4, we will get into the comprehensive practical methods for you to unleash the power of your vagus nerve. When you can fully understand how to incorporate vagal care in your daily life, you will notice many differences in your day-to-day lifestyle.

Vagus nerve stimulation could be the future of medicine. It could help treat everything from depression to Alzheimer's disease. It might be the answer for those who suffer from multiple sclerosis or frequent headaches.

We can't say for certain that this is the best treatment for these types of conditions, but we can say there is hope. Your health is one of the most precious things you'll have, and any disruption to that might start with this one nerve that runs through your body.

You might be struggling with issues with your vagus nerve if you have:

- Depression
- Anxiety
- IBS/SIBO
- Difficulty swallowing
- Chronic inflammation and fatigue
- GERD/heartburn
- Weight control problems
- Irregular sleep patterns

There are many more symptoms important to understand when discussing the vagus nerve, but these are the most common and disruptive.

The Importance of Understanding the Nerve

Welcome to the first few pages of a journey toward healing that is based on knowledge and understanding of critical systems within our body. This journey will take us through the body's autonomic nervous system (ANS)—specifically the vagus nerves—and how this nervous system impacts your health.

In looking at the role the vagus complex and its attached parasympathetic nervous system plays in autonomic bodily functions—everything that your body is taking care of subconsciously while you go about your day—you will come to understand why your body is reacting the way it is and why you're feeling the way you do.

The vagus nerve and parasympathetic nervous system form only one aspect of the autonomic systems; the other two aspects of this system are the sympathetic nervous system and the enteric nervous system (ENS).

The enteric nervous system isn't always classified as part of the autonomic nervous system—historically, it was accepted that the ANS was a dual-nervous system that remained in a tense tug-of-war, pulling one in or out of specific states. New research, including Porges Polyvagal Theory, has mapped out a deeper understanding of the complex in its entirety, and why some parts seem dormant or disconnected at times.

This book will serve as your introduction to the nerve itself, as well as its functional capabilities and the processes it uses to achieve those capabilities, and will provide guided exercises for you to practice, stimulating your nervous system to increase your health and the overall balance of your body. In coming to understand the needs your body places on this nerve, you will be able to activate it to balance out your stress and anxiety—often taxing biological responses that can leave you drained and feeling like a shadow of yourself.

We only have one body in this life, and it is our duty as its caretaker to listen to its demands and provide for its needs—otherwise, it will begin to fail. The vagus nerves form only one part of the complex puzzle that is human anatomy but provides a large support structure to enable other functionalities within the body to operate properly.

Commonly referred to as a singular, the vagus nerves branch out from the brainstem and through the abdomen, interfacing with many organs throughout the body and extending to the colon and some areas of the skin's surface. This set of nerves plays a huge role in the control of the parasympathetic nervous system—relating mostly to the abdominal organs such as the heart, lungs, and digestive tract, but also includes control of the throat and intonation. It is the backbone that this nervous system is built on, relaying messages to and from the brain to provide the correct innervation at these points.

The vagus nerve is a great communications thoroughfare, scouting reports and orders constantly firing back and forth, all to allow our lungs to breathe and our hearts to beat a rhythm of blood through our bodies in a manner that can feel effortless to us if it's in working order. A damaged vagus nerve, or at least one that is poorly stimulated, can lead to many difficulties in daily life, including problems with breathing, social interaction, blood pressure, and myriad other symptoms. Acute problems may also arise, such as vasovagal syncope, a stress-induced overreaction that often results in dizziness and fainting, and potentially gastroparesis, which causes difficulty in the body naturally removing stomach contents. This title will cover the foundation of the vagus nerve and what it does for you day in and day out, but this guide will also seek to help you heal and overcome trauma and pain associated with the vagus nerve. To do so, it is required that you have an understanding of what the nerve does to gain perspective of how the exercises in this book can affect such a delicate system and do so safely for your benefit.

The parasympathetic nervous system made up primarily of the vagus nerve, and the attached system of viscera (the body's vital organs) is one such system that can be used to affect physical change to one's body. Effects can range from bringing your blood pressure down within minutes, and it can even reduce the levels of cortisol—responsible for stress and anxiety—within your system.

The body itself works off of cues it receives from the multitude of chemical, electrical, and nervous impulses that are sent through it based on stimuli, fuel, and even alien invaders to our enclosed biological systems. Environmental cues also play a role, interpreted by our brains through our senses, and the parasympathetic system not only displays social cues for others to interpret but allows us to see and interpret those reactions in them. Remember that you don't have to go through this journey alone. Talk to your doctor before starting any intense treatment, and seek their advice in areas where you are unsure of the best approach. There is hope for those who suffer from vagus nerve-related issues, and the answers to your health conditions might be lying within these words.

Thanks for choosing this book. Enjoy your reading and if you want, leave a short review on Amazon, it's important for me!

CHAPTER 1:

THE ANATOMY OF THE VAGUS NERVE

The human body is dependent on the vagus nerve for many reasons. This system enables our lungs to breathe, ensures we swallow our food, and performs many other functions throughout the digestive tract and heart.

Extending from the medulla oblongata, the vagus nerve reaches down the same compartment as the jugular and past the pathway of main arteries to reach the surface skin of the ear, larynx, and general throat. It also extends to the organs of the cardiovascular system, and the general mass of internal organs up to the colon.

This nerve comprises a large portion of the parasympathetic nervous system and is accompanied by the sympathetic nervous system, responsible for many immediate actions due to its control over the fight-or-flight system, and the enteric nervous system (ENS), which is confined to the gastrointestinal tract and runs from end to end.

Together, these three systems make up the autonomic

nervous system:
- The parasympathetic nervous system (heart/lungs/digestion)
- The sympathetic nervous system (stress response)
- The enteric nervous system (gastrointestinal)

They are intrinsically tied to one another, often responsible for the response to the state of one system or another.

Included in the nerves' functionality are both sensory and motor actions, relating directly to communications through body language as well as control of the larynx, the rate at which our heartbeats, and the general pattern of our breathing, as well as mitigating stress levels and counteracting the fight-or-flight reaction triggered from within the amygdala. The parasympathetic nervous system is responsible for states of relaxation and is a direct counterpart to the sympathetic nervous system, which is responsible for immediate actions and is home to the amygdala.

When your body naturally calms from states of intense activity such as exercise, or even periods of stress, anger, and anxiety, it is likely due to the parasympathetic nervous kicking back in and bringing the sympathetic system back into balance with everything else.

The vagus nerves have been found responsible for directly combating levels of stress and the related hormones causing this effect, like cortisol, and through stimulation of this nerve, neurotransmitters, and enzymes are released to calm the body down. Stronger responses of this kind will provide better recovery times for a person suffering from a stressful situation, injury, or illness, and these stronger responses are found within a healthy vagus nerve.

The vagus nerve is mostly made up of sensory afferent and efferent motor nerve fibers that relay messages throughout the body, signaling responses and providing other necessary information for the body to operate. Correctly triggering these responses will induce the rest-

and-digest system within your body, causing your heart rate and blood pressure to lower as well as combating inflammation.

Intrinsic to the vagus nervous system are the secreting cells found within the nerve fibers and the smooth muscles that construct the surface of our internal organs. This network utilizes neurological responses to send and receive information each vital process in your body relies on upon, transmitting vast amounts of information at incredible speeds. The nerve endings here are also able to redirect stored energy to these areas of the body.

Structure of the Vagus Nerve

We know about the origin and general course of the nerve through the body, but this nerve impacts and innervates many systems vital to ordinary human life. In the case of malfunctioning, or even poorly functioning, vagus nerve and parasympathetic system, myriad effects will take place, or fail to, with the resulting consequence leaving an individual far less capable to handle life.

The vagus nerve is the tenth cranial nerve originating at the medulla and extending from the fourth and sixth pharyngeal arches—referring to a systematic structure of archways around the base of the brain that forms much of the foundation for the rest of its growth and structure. There are five pairs of these arches and each pair is numbered 1, 2, 3, 4, and 6, with the first three involved with the development of the head and organs above the larynx.

Within the cranium, the nerve extends to the ear to provide sensation and innervation to part of the ear canal and the exterior surface skin of the ear. From there, the branches split and enter into the throat and abdomen. In the throat, the vagus nerve plays several different roles.

The pharyngeal branches extending alongside the vagus nerve innervate most of the pharynx and soft palate, being the upper portion of your throat in direct contact with your mouth and the roof of your mouth.

Below this, the superior laryngeal nerve splits to provide somatic innervation of the muscles of the larynx and sensory innervation to the superior, or upper, larynx, as well as sensory innervation to the laryngopharynx (the connection between the larynx and pharynx, being a part of the pharynx itself).

The recurrent laryngeal nerve (found only on the right side of the body) plays a role in the larynx, despite the circuitous route it takes. This nerve extends from the original vagus nerve farther down the throat and hooks underneath an artery before climbing back up to the larynx to innervate many of the smaller muscles found in the throat.

At this juncture, the vagus muscle has specific control over airflow, as well as the vocal box. Furthermore, this is the entry point for food into our gastrointestinal tract, and the nerve controls and assists the intake of food at the entry point of the pharynx and larynx, utilizing the epiglottis to this end.

From here, the nerve continues into the main body cavity and over the esophagus creating the esophageal plexus, which innervates the smooth muscles found within the esophagus, continuing the close ties the vagus nerve has to the gastrointestinal tract and intrinsic nature of the vagus nerve regarding the control and management of digestion.

The nerve branches again, extending out toward the heart and providing innervation of the myocardium, which allows the nerve to regulate the heartbeat and provide sensation to the organ.

From here, the nerve enters its final length as it branches out along the esophagus, around the stomach and intestines. The nerve provides innervation to these organs as well as visceral sensations. As part of the vagal system, the vagus can provide small amounts of food and fuel throughout its network to the organs it supplies, as well as carrying other nutrients and enzymes to other connected systems.

Given how intertwined the vagus nerve is with much of one's internal organs, the extensive surface area of the viscera, and the nature of efferent nerves—being that of carrying information—it is clear that extensive sensory data is carried across this system. As large as it is, the gut may be an important organ in this function given its size, and more so especially when considering it processes the most information from the outside world across its vast surface within this system.

Alongside providing all of this information and relaying these messages back and forth, the vagus nerve is the backbone, additionally, to the parasympathetic nervous system and everything that entails—in regards directly to the digestive system, rest, and many of the subconscious actions our organs are responsible for. The parasympathetic system is directly responsible for lowering the rate of one's heart through the release of acetylcholine—which is also a crucial factor in the breathing process—and the dilation of blood vessels. The vagus system supplies a range of other signals to release enzymes and proteins such as prolactin, vasopressin, and oxytocin, or even to counteract the production of some enzymes relating to glucose such as Phosphoenolpyruvate carboxykinase and Glucose 6-phosphatase, which are produced in the liver.

In contrast to the parasympathetic nervous system, the sympathetic counterpart is responsible for action—priming the muscles, heart, and lungs, all in the aim of preparing the body to move and engage. The sympathetic draws blood away from the end goal of its counterpart, being the gut and adjacent organ, and up to the cardiovascular bodies. The sympathetic system will also prime muscles the body deems necessary to answer what has triggered the response in conjunction with the amygdala and the fight-or-flight instinct.

As part of its role in transitioning into the resting stage, the vagus nerve will release enzymes directly into the amygdala to turn off its response and immediately reduce the production of the stress hormone. A healthy vagus nerve will provide a quicker transition and more appropriate response to high levels of cortisol dumped into the system.

As part of the vegetative functions of one's body, the vagus nerve is directly intertwined with the enteric nervous system and together plays many vital roles within the control of eating, swallowing, bowel mobility, sleeping, and sexual arousal and performance.

The Brain-Gut Axis

The connection between the brain and the gut is commonly described as the brain-gut axis due to its role relaying information from the enteric nervous system to the central nervous system (CNS) and vice-versa. At the juncture at which these systems meet, it additionally allows control of the function of the intestines and nutrient absorption, as well as the activation of the immune system. Each system plays a role in the combined function, and only in its healthy function will it be allowed to work properly with the other systems.

This brain-gut axis is made up of the brain itself, the spinal cord, the autonomic nervous system, which includes the various nervous systems mentioned and the hormonal axis—this is constructed by the connection of the hypothalamic, adrenal, and pituitary glands (HPA axis). These links are crucial as the HPA axis is responsible for acting on stressors on the body, involving the vagal nerve pathway running to the brain, and triggers the release of cytokines and the corticotropin-releasing factor (CRF) secreted from the hypothalamus. This, in turn, triggers the pituitary gland to release the adrenocorticotropic hormone (ACTH) through secretion and finally allows the adrenal gland to join in by providing cortisol, the main stress hormone that has major effects on the structure of the body.

This system is further influenced by gut microbiota (ecological communities of certain microorganisms) that are responsible for the balance and state of the microbial environment within the stomach.

A recent study set out to implicate the treatment or prevention of some psychological illnesses, such as depression and anxiety, through different approaches regarding the gastrointestinal microbiota, dietary plans, and other possible avenues. The study helped show a balanced microbiome can occur naturally due to the colonization of intestinal microbiota. The bacteria along the gastrointestinal tract helps to stimulate important signals within the central nervous system.

The vagal system and the microbiota are further dependent on one another as the afferents leading from the vagus nerves and innervating the gastrointestinal tract provide nutrients and circulate store fuels within a discrete amount. Vagal efferent running back up the system is influenced by the hormonal axis, determining rates of nutritional absorption, mobility, and cases of storage (Field, Chaudhri, & Bloom, 2012).

Health Implications of the Vagus Nerve

The system that we are currently exploring has been shown to provide for a variety of basic needs within our body and the unique systems therein. Your nervous system supports diverse functions ranging from control of the throat, voice box, and esophagus—and generally playing a massive role in the digestive tract—to allowing and regulating the function of the heart.

This system can also implicate everything that it is involved in, including the brain-gut and hormonal axes, leading to systems losing functionality or becoming hyperactive. The impact of a damaged or unhealthy vagus nerve can even extend beyond this system to impact the enteric nervous system as well as the central nervous system, creating complications with senses and moods.

Digestion is greatly impacted by a stressed vagal system

and can even lead to complications in answering the call of nature, specifically in emptying stomach contents.

Other symptoms and complications can arise that are direr and more pressing than a full colon, such as arrhythmic heart rates, inefficient oxygen supply to vital areas of the body, and comprised blood supply as the body reacts incorrectly and draws blood from the functions that need it.

In serious cases a condition called vasovagal syncope arises, which causes your blood pressure to drop rapidly at specific stress triggers—these can include the sight of blood, emotional duress, and more.

These are not the only effects that a compromised vagus nerve can have on the body, as a vagal nerve that is presenting in an unnatural state directly affects the other parts of the autonomic nervous system, being the sympathetic nervous system and the enteric nervous system, as the parasympathetic system the vagus nerve controls is key to balancing out these other systems.

Considering the Significance of Emotional Health with the Vagus Nerve

The vagus nerves play a key role in stabilizing mood, mostly by providing chemical counterparts that slow or inhibit the effects of other chemicals in our body—examples of these chemicals are cortisol and cytokines.

The vagal system is specifically engineered to bring the body back into balance, to a calm and restive state, while autonomically handling core bodily functions necessary to our survival. Within this, the vagal tone plays a key role and is a measurement that can indicate the current state of the vagus nerves. This refers to the rate of the heart, generally at rest, and the difference in time between pumping blood out and back in.

It has been shown that a healthy vagal tone is responsible for the ability to manage stress and stress triggers within the body. The ability to do so is closely linked with the brain-gut axis mentioned above and the interaction with the hormonal axis. The activity within the vagus nerve correlates greatly to the influence of moods and psychiatric disorders along the lines of anxiety and depression.

Stimulation of the vagus nerve is thought to contribute to the body's natural defenses against these disorders and bring a general sense of well-being and balance back to oneself.

CHAPTER 2:

THE FUNCTIONS OF THE VAGUS NERVE

Innervation—providing organs or other parts of the body with nerve endings—is one major capacity of the vagus nerve within the body. While the vagus nerve is the body's longest cranial nerve and it does branch off throughout the throat, abdomen, and around other organs, it specifically provides these nerve endings to the gastrointestinal tract and many related organs, as well as a few unrelated that remain close to the pathway of the vagus nerve, as we described in the previous chapter.

An aspect of innervation provides sensation to the innervated organs or constructs and providing them with a network to communicate the sensations they feel back to the brain, as well as relaying information to any necessary nervous action centers. To do so, the nerves are broken down into afferent endings and efferent endings. The communications sent along these pathways are dedicated to one direction.

Afferent nerves are sensory neural pathways that carry impulses from stimuli and input back up your nervous system and to your brain. The message is processed and interpreted and sent back out to efferent nerves.

Efferent nerves are motor neurons that send signals back out to the relevant part of the body, based on the interpretation of need from the brain, and cause the body to react. Efferent nerves exit the spinal cord near various groups of muscles so that any reaction can be transmitted directly to a select group of tissue.

As an example, if you were to cut your hand on something sharp, the immediate sensation is of the tissue slicing open as well as the accompanying pain, and perhaps a bit of heat from the blood and inflammation—that message is all relayed to the brain through afferent nerves along with the nervous system. Your brain interprets this as a danger, as you already have sustained a wound, and will send signals along the efferent neural pathways and out to the motor processes of the body to affect the necessary actions to bring your body away from the danger and, perhaps, even to defend yourself from harm.

If there is no further threat, especially in the case of a nick from your knife as you sliced through a tomato, the parasympathetic system will kick in to calm the body down, and the next outcome is to assess the damage and go about tending the wound. The sensation from the wound allows your body to tell itself, and you, more about it by relaying the pain from the affected tissue and back to the brain. These sensations are also afferent and will lead to efferent communication as you seek medical attention.

The vagus nerve provides this combination of sensory input and active output to the organs and structures that it innervates, mostly providing visceral sensation and control to the body.

Sensory Functionality Provided by the Vagus Nerve

The sensory function of the vagus nerve is mainly communicative in sending the appropriate signals from the origin of stimuli to the central nervous system and brain, and out again to the body. This is broken up into two separate forms of function, that being visceral (relating to the organs) and somatic (relating to the skin and muscles).

Somatic Innervation of the Vagus Nerve

The somatic function of the vagus nerve is centralized in the cranium, specifically around the ear, through communication with the auricular nerve. The auricular branch of the vagus nerve, extending from the superior ganglion of this nerve, provides innervation of the skin within the ear canal as well as the exterior of the ear.

Dysfunction of this branch of the vagus can cause complications with the function and senses of the affected aspects of the ear. Additionally, sensitivity in the area can cause stimulation to elicit a cough, known as an Ear-Cough, from a particular subject. In some exceptional cases, distress caused in the patient by inserting an object such as a speculum, which is used to explore the body's orifices and create space to better allow investigation, or an otoscope, a simple tool used in a general checkup of the ear by allowing the doctor a direct, unobstructed and illuminated view of the ear canal, can present as fainting in patients.

It has been proposed that "transcutaneous vagus nerve stimulation" (tVNS), achieved through external stimulation of the terminal nerve endings attached to the vagus nerve by methods such as massaging the surface, can provide therapeutic treatment for seizures as a method of control and prevention (Ventureya, 2000). Later, other researchers compiled further studies associated with the outcomes of tVNS and the variegated conditions stimulation of this nerve may affect.

In 2003, Fallgatter et al. produced the paper "Far-Field Potentials from the Brain Stem After Transcutaneous Vagus Nerve Stimulation," which expounded upon the original assertations of Ventureya, and went on to further detail the role neurodegenerative diseases such as Alzheimer's impact the basic structure of the vagus nerve early in their course.

Several years down the line, a study was conducted utilizing functional magnetic resonance imaging (fMRI) that tracks the blood flow within the brain to map the activity of the cerebral tissue (BOLD fMRI Deactivation of Limbic and Temporal Brain Structures and Mood Enhancing Effect by Transcutaneous Vagus Nerve Stimulation, 2007). At this point, direct vagus nerve stimulation (dVNS) had proven itself a worthwhile treatment for disorders involving seizures as well as major depressions—stimulation of the vagus nerve has shown to affect and treat depressive disorders that cannot adequately be handled by antidepressants—but the title of 'direct' stimulation implies surgery of some kind.

The team of Kraus et al. set out to prove that tVNS is viable as a form of treatment for these same disorders, but without any invasive procedure. The study found that brain activation under tVNS produced similar patterns to a brain under dVNS, meriting that transcutaneous stimulation of the vagus nerve could become a mainstream add-on treatment for several conditions, if not the direct cure itself.

Visceral Innervation of the Vagus Nerve

Alongside the somatic responsibilities of the vagus nerve, it is also intrinsically tied to the organs in our main body cavities. Visceral innervation begins within the throat at the laryngopharynx and the muscles of the larynx. These pharyngeal and laryngeal branches supply motor impulses to the pharynx and larynx, allowing constriction and control of these areas, as well as providing the necessary action to vocalize. Sensations of pain and discomfort will be sent as signals from the origins at this point along the same branches and back to the brain.

The vagus continues to innervate organs as it enters into the thorax and abdomen, specifically branching to provide for cardiac and pulmonary functions around the heart and lungs. The function of the vagus at this point to control the rate at which the heartbeats, in addition to the constriction of the bronchi within the conductive system in the lungs.

Issues can arise at this point through a dysfunctional

vagus nerve by presenting in arrhythmical heartbeats, cardiac infarctions, tightness of chest, and difficulty breathing. Stress triggers can cause the chest cavity and lungs to seize until the sympathetic nervous system releases its hold on the body.

Visceral innervation is crucial to the health, function, and structure of the gastrointestinal tract, playing a role from the top of the system down to its termination. The branch of the vagus directly affecting this area allows control of the involuntary muscles for the gut, gallbladder, small and large intestines, esophagus, and pancreas. Control of these areas will signal the wave-like motion (peristalsis) starting at the top of the gastrointestinal tract that begins upon ingesting food and allowing it to travel to the stomach—and again, it is crucial in the management and removal of waste as it travels through the colon. The vagus nerve also signals gastrointestinal secretions that fire along this pathway to assist in the breakdown and absorption of nutrients, as well as removing waste products with discretion.

Parasympathetic Role of the Vagus Nerve Within the Heart and Gastrointestinal Tract

Parasympathetic nerve endings stem from the cardiac branches of the vagus nerve to interface with the heart. This system is constantly firing to maintain a resting heartbeat of around 60 to 80 beats per minute or to bring the heart rate from an active rate to the rate of rest.

A lesioned vagus nerve can lead to an increase of the resting heart rate, pushing the upper bound to 100 beats per minute or above. This is not the only risk involved within the parasympathetic nervous system and the heart, as arrhythmic heartbeats can become a constant risk to your daily health. A damaged vagus nerve can lead to other conditions affecting the parasympathetic system and can be as devastating as cardiac infarction.

Within the gastrointestinal tract, the vagus nerve provides parasympathetic innervation directly to smooth muscles of the viscera to allow for the contraction of these muscles as well as signaling for chemical secretion within the organs. Improper signaling can cause complications within each of these systems individually.

Special Sensory Function of the Vagus Nerve

While the vagus nerve does provide sensation from other organs within the body, it is mostly concerned without touch, pain, inflammation, and discomfort. A minor role of the vagus nerve outside of these phenomena is specifically concerned with the root of the tongue and the epiglottis.

Afferent nerve endings are provided from the vagus nerve to allow a taste sensation in those particular oral constructs.

Motor Functions in the Pharynx and Larynx

With very few exceptions, the vagus nerve is responsible for providing motor signaling and control within the throat. The motor functions are split to affect the pharynx and the larynx separately, providing different responsibilities to each area in the throat.

Much of what the vagus does within the throat involves initiating swallowing and the function of peristalsis, as well as phonation associated with speech. Additionally, as usual, the vagus nerve is responsible for relaying communications about pain and inflammation from this area to the brain.

Motorized Innervation of the Pharynx

Much of the pharynx is solely innervated by the pharyngeal branches of the vagus nerve, excepting for the Stylopharyngeus muscle (concerned mostly with elevating the larynx and pharynx) which is innervated by the glossopharyngeal nerve, or ninth cranial nerve. This process creates more space in the throat and directly dilates the pharynx to allow larger amounts of food to pass through. This process facilitates swallowing but takes place beforehand.

Beyond this, the vagus nerve further innervates the salpingopharyngeal muscle, which assists with both speaking and swallowing by shortening the pharynx and raising the larynx. Additionally, this muscle controls the opening of the Eustachian (auditory) tube within the pharyngeal construct.

Motorized Innervation of the Larynx

Breaking down the innervation of the larynx will split it over the innervation provided by the differing laryngeal branches of the vagus nerve.

The simplest function and innervation of this grouping seem to be that of the external laryngeal nerve. This nerve branch interfaces with the cricothyroid muscle, being the only tensor muscle (preoccupied with the tightening or stretching of a particular area of the body) that aids in the act of phonation by tensing the vocal cords. This nerve is often confused with the posterior cricoarytenoid muscles, which open the space between the vocal cords to allows air to pass through—the cricothyroid muscle group has no role to play in respiration.

The recurrent laryngeal nerve—named so as it loops down under an aorta and ascends back to the larynx—is responsible for myriad systems within the throat and larynx. This particular network does control the posterior cricoarytenoid muscle group, alongside that of the lateral cricoarytenoid, and transverse and oblique arytenoid muscle groups. Each of these muscle groups plays a role in opening or closing the throat to allow both a food bolus or air to pass through, and at times closing off the channel of this pathway as other actions fire off further down the network.

The vocalis and thyroarytenoid muscles that form part of this construct are directly involved in forming the vocal cords into the correct formation to produce phonation. The vocalis directly affects the thickness of the vocal cords, whereas the thyroarytenoid is a complicated system that moves cartilage forward to relax and shorten the vocal folds.

Beyond this, the vagus nerve provides innervation to the palatoglossus, responsible for raising the rear section of the tongue, and much of the muscles within the soft palate.

Hoarseness and Difficulty Swallowing Associated with the Vagus Nerve

Given the intricate nature of the vagus nerve, as well as the associated and specialized systems the nerve allows functionality to, it is not hard to understand that a compromised vagus nerve will directly impact the efficacy of all systems within this network.

The laryngeal branches of the vagus nerve are no strangers to restrictions, nor are they impervious to damage. The recurrent vagus nerve can easily be constricted underneath the aorta it loops around, producing hoarseness in the voice most commonly associated with laryngitis. Additional forms of damage can impact the voice in other manners, and these forms of damage can also create difficulty in swallowing or creating the necessary space for unobstructed airflow.

Physical Implications on the Body Caused by Complications in the Vagus Nerve

The vagus nerve and parasympathetic nervous systems are both diverse and far-reaching within the human body. The vagus nerve provides for many vital and basic systems of survival for any human being, as well as playing the counterpart to calming the sympathetic nervous system. Further diversified are the specific functions of the muscle groups and organs in which the nerve-endings of the vagus terminate.

This system is complicated and intricate, and it's easy to see how a small change can have a huge impact. Factors of input, ranging from sensory input and internal signaling, to intake, such as diet and nutrition, can have a radical impact on the functionality of the vagus nerve and the associated system. Stressors on the vagus nerve can also heavily impact the entire network, especially under improper and obtuse response from the vagus nerve.

Some of the serious complications that can arise are fainting through vasovagal syncope or the over-stimulation of the vagal system through stress and sensory overload, as well as a paralysis within the process of emptying food from the stomach in a regular manner.

Vasovagal Syncope

When triggered, vasovagal syncope causes both your blood pressure and heart rate to plummet suddenly. Upon doing so, stress is placed on vital parts of the anatomy, constricting blood from through the heart and to the brain, and this deprivation of oxygenated blood can lead to a fainting spell.

Internal symptoms of vasovagal syncope occur shortly before the fainting spell. The symptoms you should be alert for include pale skin (a sign of restricted blood flow), lightheadedness, nausea, cold and clammy sweat, as well as tunnel vision, blurred vision, or even a TV-like static from the days of cathode-ray tubes. Vision can become completely filled with constantly shifting black, white, and grey spots.

Any onlooker in these cases might see abnormal and jerky motion and dilated pupils, along with the sensation of a weakened pulse under inspection. Recovery begins within a minute a two, but rising too rapidly from a spell of vasovagal syncope may induce the same result again.

Instead, collect yourself and breathe—this will bring the parasympathetic nervous system back under your control and normalize the levels within this system.

The biological reaction under this stress is that the blood vessels in the legs dilate, causing blood to pool low in the extremities of the body. This lowers the heart rate and reduces effective blood flow to the brain, and makes it more difficult for the nervous system to maintain rigid muscles. Ultimately, a combination of these effects will result in blacking out.

There is no specific trigger that is always present in vasovagal syncope, but the condition can be triggered through standing for extended durations (allowing blood to naturally pool in the legs), through exposure to heat, excessively straining the body through physical activity, or any process involving exposed blood or having it drawn from the body.

If you suffer from any fainting spell, it is advisable to seek professional medical advice as this symptom may be a result of a more serious condition.

Gastroparesis

This is a condition of the gut generally caused by damage to the vagus nerve. The role of the vagus nerve implicated here is that of contracting the muscles of the gut to allow the movement of food through the gastrointestinal tract. Under stress or through damage, the control of these muscles is undermined, and it is difficult to move food and waste throughout the remainder of the digestive tract.

Other complications that can lead to this same cause are viral infections or any gastric surgery that caused damage to the vagus nerve (this also includes a vagotomy, a procedure in which branches of the vagus nerve are intentionally cut to provide treatment for other conditions), and certain medications such as narcotics and antidepressants can present this as a side-effect.

The symptoms of this condition include heartburn, nausea, vomiting of undigested food, feeling full early in instances of eating, bloating of the stomach and abdomen, as well as a poor appetite that is associated with unnatural weight loss.

Generally, the damage to the vagus nerve that causes this issue is derived from the acute disorder of diabetes, directly affecting the brain-gut axis due to the improper regulation of bodily sugars.

The complications of this disorder vary but can include the fermentation of food within the stomach, leading to unnatural and increased rates of bacterial growth.

Bezoars, solids masses of food, can form by hardening within the stomach itself. Bezoars lead to multiple complications, including the restriction of the gut and the possibility of blockages created at the juncture of the stomach and the intestine. Bezoars can be painful, but they also impact the capacity of food intact as well as the ability to process that food.

Gastroparesis can cause additional complications in that when the food finally enters the rest of the digestive tract, it can lead to a rapid escalation in the levels of glucose. This can be further complicated by the condition of diabetes, as well as presenting in additional complications due to the unstable levels of glucose in the body.

Dehydration and malnutrition become a factor in gastroparesis as the nutrition locked within the food substances fail to reach the necessary area to provide a wash of nutrients or even water. Any form of nutritional absorption primarily takes place within the intestines, and gastroparesis is the bouncer holding the line at the door.

to process that food.

Gastroparesis can cause additional complications in that when the food finally enters the rest of the digestive tract, it can lead to a rapid escalation in the levels of glucose. This can be further complicated by the condition of diabetes, as well as presenting in additional complications due to the unstable levels of glucose in the body.

Dehydration and malnutrition become a factor in gastroparesis as the nutrition locked within the food substances fail to reach the necessary area to provide a wash of nutrients or even water. Any form of nutritional absorption primarily takes place within the intestines, and gastroparesis is the bouncer holding the line at the door.

CHAPTER 3:

THE POLYVAGAL THEORY

Originating in 1995, the polyvagal theory is the brainchild of Stephen Porges. Porges utilized clinical study and observations from both the side of evolutionary biology or phylogenesis, as well as general neurology, before propagating the (at the time) newly discovered connection of the vagus nerve and parasympathetic nervous system containing an afferent network that drew signals to the brain.

Much of the polyvagal theory is based on the physical construct of the vagus nerve and its role as the foundation of the function of the parasympathetic nervous system, but it also pairs the extent of the parasympathetic nervous system with that of the sympathetic.

Established in his original work on the vagus nerve, Porges identified that the parasympathetic system was a direct counterpart, or even control, of the sympathetic system, and spoke about how the vagal systems play a crucial role in reacting appropriately to danger alongside the sympathetic-adrenal connection.

Porges proposed the vagus is split along two distinct branches based on phylogenetic evidence collected not only from human biology but that of various other animals as well. For Porges, the vagus was ultimately a complex structure that developed new characteristics and functions as human biology evolved, and the latter, more complex systems take precedence in control of the body's functions and the former, basic evolutionary systems only kick in once action or response from the higher systems has failed.

Foundation of the Polyvagal Theory and the Dichotomous Branch System

The two networks within the vagus were proposed as the dorsal vagal complex or DVC, and the ventral vagal complex, or VVC, of which the DVC is considered older, phylogenetically. This complex has been observed in most vertebrates.

The dorsal vagal complex originates from the dorsal motor nucleus of the vagus and can be found in the medulla. This system is integral to most viscera within the body, providing control and innervation to the organs found below the diaphragm. The DVC has also become known as the "vegetative vagus" due to its implicit nature in addition to its association with primal instincts relevant to survival.

The DVC serves as a network to handle various stress responses within mammals. A major function of the dorsal vagal complex in survival relates to shutting down the body, an attempt to play dead or limit the biological signs of life such as heart rate. This reaction is triggered under immense levels of stress or when faced with threats and it attempts to preserve the metabolic functions of the creature.

This form of disinhibition can lead to other complications and dangers within some mammals, such as difficulty in regulating one's heartbeat and even apnea, the disruption of breathing due to the muscles associated with inhalation not activating.

Due to complexities arising from an ever-changing environment and social structure development, the mammalian neural system generated a new system to work alongside the dorsal vagal complex—that being the ventral vagal complex, directly tied to the functionality of the organs residing above the diaphragm. This branch originates in the nucleus ambiguous (quite literally the ambiguous nucleus) found in the structure of the medulla and gives rise to expanded responses through the behavioral and efferent systems.

Unlike the dorsal vagal complex, the ventral vagal complex is sheathed in a fatty layer—called myelin—that, under attachment to nerve cells, creates an insulating layer for those cells. In addition to this, the physical makeup of the myelin allows the nerve to better conduct stimulus through its system by allowing electrical impulses to pass through at a rapidly increased rate. Myelinated nerve cells are the quickest to respond and, ultimately, provide more control than their unmyelinated counterparts. The myelin sheath is most commonly associated with later evolutionary development to assist in more complicated systems as human civilization grew.

Part of this responsibility comes to the fore as the ventral vagal complex acts to regulate the sympathetic nervous system and to suppress overreactions within that system to better support behaviors associated with socialization. Included in these services is the ability of social communication, which involves clearly expressing yourself to another individual as well as correctly interpreting their self-expression, as well as bodily systems that allow one to soothe and calm themselves.

The ventral vagus complex has a strong connection to the heart and lungs through efferent nerve cells that stem from the nerve cells that originate in the nucleus ambiguous. Part of this complex contains motor neurons, allowing for physical control over the action of these organs, but also parasympathetic cells that assist in modulating their function. From this network, the vagus can determine whether to inhibit action derived from the limbic circuits or to remove the inhibition and allow mobilization and action more easily.

This pattern of inhibition and disinhibition is continued in the ventral vagal complex as a vagal tone.

The tone assists in the pacemaker functions of the heart. The vagus nerve and parasympathetic nervous system act to lower the heart rate, and it is due to the VVC providing a limit on the rate of the heart.

This influence over the heart directly affects one's ability to respond to danger. A healthy vagal tone and a correctly functioning parasympathetic system allow all the necessary corresponding systems to engage in turn, but it also modulates these responses to maintain general stability. An excessive reaction in either direction can become damaging to the body, especially as any engagement of the sympathetic-adrenal system can come with a severe biological cost.

Interestingly enough, once vagal tone has been removed from the equation, inhibition on the heart and its pacemaker become greatly lessened—to a point where the same communications to move can be generated without the reliance of the fight-or-flight system.

Prolonged exposure to disinhibition of the vagal complexes can lead to health complications arising in associated and peripheral systems, and this disorder can become lethal through health complications if left unchecked. This can include an arrhythmic heart rate, as well as difficulties and obstructions in breathing.

Miscellaneous Cases of the Impact a Damaged Vagus Nerve can Cause the Brain

Myriad clinical studies on the vagus nerve have shown a variety of psychiatric implications and applications of the vagus nerve. The irrefutable evidence of these has been discussed above, but before these conditions made it into psychiatric practice, they were poorly understood or completely miscategorized.

The same can be said for incipient understandings that are now being found and cataloged as new cases and clinical studies are put forward. On the fringes of our knowledge of the vagus nerve and other physiological entities, new questions are arising. The more knowledge we turn over, it appears, the more questions we find among the answers.

Some lesser documented affects the vagus nerve can have on the brain include the role it would play in the formation of memories, as well as sustained damage from mental abuse, in the case of narcissistic abuse.

Homeostasis and the Vagal Tone

Homeostasis is a balance created within the body that is controlled by the various systems within said body. This provides steady conditions that relate to the body's chemical and physical states, dynamically changing as the body's demands change—this is affected by the central nervous system reacting to the current environmental situation as well as cues provided by sensory organs.

Stressful incidents disrupt the rest and digestion system, breaking the parasympathetic response and changing the behavioral response triggered by environmental cues. Physiologically, this is experienced as an increase in the respiratory sinus arrhythmia (RSA)—being the change in respiratory rhythm that maintains a shortened pattern on inhalation and reflecting a prolonged duration on exhalation—and can be measured non-invasively through machines such as an ECG. This has given rise to measuring vagal tone and parasympathetic activity through the measurement of the RSA.

Through research, it has been shown that amplitude in the RSA is the best current indicator for any outgoing influence of the vagus nerve on the heart, being modulation of and reduction in the rate of the heart through inhibition. This can be used to determine individual reactions to stress as well as possible abnormalities in the body relating to stress and the reaction to stress.

Beyond this, the inhibitory effects of the ventral vagal complex and their association with expanded social and adaptive behaviors have led researchers to posit that those with a higher vagal tone are capable of a wider range of associated behaviors, but additionally, they can adapt and react more appropriately to stress. Unfortunately, on the opposite end of the spectrum, complications (such as mood affective disorders) can lead to limited social exposure and interaction due to compromised neural pathways. Additionally, a low vagal tone creates an internal environment that is limited or incapable of appropriately reacting to stress.

Vagal tone, specifically referring to the activity of the vagus nerve, has correlated to many health-boosting and positive effects within one's body. A healthy vagal tone is generally strong and plays several roles in regulating the body's systems and condition. Often, this can be measured through heart-rate variability—the minor rhythmic changes between each beat—but this method does not provide accurate results.

A healthy vagal tone also allows for the regulation of the sympathetic nervous system and other aspects of the body. Without keeping these systems in check, imbalances begin to arise within the human body—and complications are soon to follow.

The implication of the vagus nerve on mood and similar disorders is mostly derived from its capacity within the HPA axis, the mediation and control directly opposing the sympathetic nervous system and limbic system, as well as its role within the brain-gut access and the influence of the microbiota within. This network provides the body with the infrastructure to transport and provide the various enzymes, hormones, and chemicals that form part of these functions.

Additionally, the production of these specific chemicals can be halted or increased through stimulation within the vagus nerve and related systems.

Given this nature of the vagus, it is clear to see that the nerve is integral to the modulation of one's mood and general emotional stability. Beyond this, stimulation of the vagus nerve has been observed to directly impact the negative effects of brain fog, physical and mental fatigue, anxious mood disorders, depressive disorders and episodes alongside digestive stress by strengthening your vagal tone.

Several options of therapeutic treatment, especially for dysfunction and disorder directly relating to the vagus nerve and parasympathetic system, can be found through different options of stimulating the vagus nerve. These actions are intrinsically tied to the bodily functions of the related systems the vagus nerve innervates, such as holding your breath or meditating.

Polyvagal Theory in Practice

Trauma occurs to more people than we realize, and it consistently derives responses from us driven from the threats we perceive. Before discovering the polyvagal theory, it was believed there were just two simple reactions created in the vagus nerve:

- Fight/flight (sympathetic)
- Freeze/faint (parasympathetic)

The polyvagal theory introduces the third reaction, what Porges refers to as the social engagement system. We discussed in this chapter the basic anatomy of these structures, but now let's get a better idea of how they practically apply to our life.

We all have to socially interact as humans. We must get to know other people and share common ideas with them for consistent growth. The reactions and responses we have toward the actions of others can cause us personal distress and even traumatic experiences.

Whatever trauma you endured as a child will show through how you interact with those around you now. If you were constantly bullied and made to feel like a nobody, you might struggle to find confidence. If you were raised in a hostile environment, you likely struggled because you were always on the defense, ready to attack anyone who threatened your views or ideas.

This kind of response carries with you today. If you perceive someone is judging your character, perhaps you're quick to lash out on them, or unable to accept criticism.

The polyvagal theory explains the idea that the balance between those responses is continuously being monitored to drive our levels of calmness or stimulation. Think of it like the way you drive a car. You don't press on the gas the entire time—you press, let up, press, and so on. If you're using cruise control, the car maintains the speed on its own, but there is some slowing and speeding when managed by yourself.

An unbalanced vagal nerve might result in that freeze response when unwarranted, or maybe you are ready to 'fight' and become aggressive when it's not necessary. By using therapy based around the polyvagal theory, you can elicit the essential balance for proper social interaction.

The polyvagal theory in therapy assists to help the patient re-pattern pathways within the nervous system. When practically applied, it enables the patient to look at the way they cope and manage their mental disorders, trauma, and anxiety, and switch those patterned ideas to something more productive and helpful.

Those who seek these kinds of therapies can use the help of a trained therapist to elicit proper vagus stimulation. This would involve:

- Deep breathing
- Light therapy
- Art expression

Another form of therapy is meditation and yoga, both of which will be covered later in the book. We will dive deeper into these methods so you can begin your therapy, or include this practice in addition to professional therapy.

We are shifting now from the more scientific part of the book to the emotional aspect. Rather than anatomy, we will focus on feeling. Instead of studying biological structures, we are going to help you implement practical strategies to unleash the power of your vagus nerve. This is something that is constantly working without your knowledge, and it's essential to take control.

Psychiatric Significance

Stimulation of a healthy vagus nerve can be effective in aiding with psychiatric conditions such as:

- PTSD
- Depressive disorders
- Anxiety-based disorders

It's important to note that seeking professional treatment alongside your self-practice efforts is always encouraged. Of course, it's not a requirement, but it can have significant effects on your recovery.

Without you even thinking about it, your vagus nerve is ensuring that you are prepared for whatever comes your way. No matter what threat is perceived, it is up to your vagus nerve to react properly. This has many physical effects, as we discussed, but most importantly, it can affect your psychology.

Your stomach might be out of balance, your heart might beat too fast too often, and you might struggle with your breathing. While this might be the biggest issue you're hoping to overcome, you'll also discover that they can all be related back to your anxiety, depression, and trauma.

These mental illnesses are often patterns that appear in our lives. Triggers keep us feeling anxious and it's challenging to overcome the worrying thoughts. These often appear as cognitive distortions.

A cognitive distortion is any repetition of the same kind

of thoughts on a repeated basis. These are usually negative or unhealthy thoughts but are often perceived as normal based on their frequency. Common cognitive distortions include:

- Black and white thinking (all or nothing)
- Absolute phrasing (best/worst, always/never, can't/shouldn't)
- Catastrophizing (I lost my job so I am going to die!)
- Personalization (The people in the corner are laughing at me)
- Jumping to conclusions (No one is coming to my party so I'm not going to have one)

The balance that is maintained by the vagus nerve can send reactions to your brain based on these responses evoked from the situations you are in.

If you hear those people laughing in the corner at a party and think that they are mocking you, it sends signals to your brain to create defenses.

This can lead to anxious thoughts at the party, sending you home early. You can go into a depressive state or even relive trauma from a moment when you were bullied in high school by a different group of laughing students.

By controlling those reactions, you're stimulating your vagus nerve to be calm in the situation. It can be challenging at first, but that nerve balance can be discovered through the right kinds of treatment.

Physical Symptoms of Mental Health Disorders

Think of your vagus nerve as the highway between your brain and your body. What happens to one is going to happen to the other.

Right now, your nerve might be clogged and congested. There's a two-hour backup worse than the traffic in L.A.

Once information gets sent to your brain, it can begin to react in more ways than just turning back for a round trip. If the pathway isn't totally clear, mixed messages will be sent to your body, those signals are lost in the wrong places, and things can get ugly.

Anxiety and depression are common, with millions of sufferers all over the world—and those are only reported numbers. No one can guess how many are silently suffering or unaware that their thought processes are abnormal.

We all have stress. Stress is extremely normal and can be helpful in certain situations. It might motivate you to get out of bed in the morning and power through at work. Stress can help us find solutions and it can make us act quickly in demanding scenarios.

Unmanaged stress can be extremely damaging, however. It can lead to frequent anxiety, to the point that you're stressed out at everything you endure.

Chronic anxiety can leave us feeling overwhelmed. You might have constant cognitive distortions. Among patterned thoughts, you could also feel:

- Fast breathing
- Sharp chest pain
- Shaking
- Tingling
- Panic/worry

Those with unmanaged anxiety can also suffer from depression, and the imbalance can cause constant mood swings and panic.

Depression is characterized by a lack of:

- Energy
- Emotion
- Self-esteem
- Focus

Depression can lead to a decrease in the production of regulatory hormones, like serotonin. The polyvagal theory essentially explains that this disruption in the hormonal balance of one's body is brought about by the regulation of the vagus nerve. When it's stimulated at the wrong time, it sends signals that cause chaos in the brain.

This can lead to physical symptoms, such as:

- Headaches
- Sore jaw
- Neck/back pain
- Constant sweating
- Teeth grinding
- Tense muscles
- Restless legs

The hormonal imbalance we discussed through the gut-brain connection can lead you to have digestive issues. It might cause frequent gas, painful bowel movements, and over or under eating.

Throughout the next four chapters of this book, we're going to help you unlock the ways you can begin to rebalance your vagus nerve to avoid these consistent negative symptoms.

Narcissistic Abuse

Narcissistic abuse is characterized by undue emotional stress in the specific context of an important person in your life—a parental figure, a friend, or even a companion—minimizing your feelings and needs while prioritizing their own. The narcissist is a particularly selfish person that uses many sociopathic patterns of behavior to manipulate you into providing for their demands.

Often, someone with a narcissistic personality disorder will hide behind their emotional manipulation and attempt to spin the situation on the person they are currently victimizing, making it out to be that the victim is, in fact, the narcissist and that their behavior is unfair. The narcissist specifically intends for the victim to question themselves while lowering their self-worth, isolating them from healthy relationships, and overall dominating the life of the victim.

While narcissistic abuse doesn't directly impact the vagus nerve or the parasympathetic system (to our knowledge), it does affect the adjacent sympathetic nervous system, and in doing so upsets the balance of autonomic system due to states of emotional duress forcing the brain out of its optimal range of the function.

Memory Creation

Memory is an important part of life. It's helpful to remember things like phone and social security numbers. Life's simpler when you can recall tasty recipes or the lyrics to your favorite songs. Life has meaning when we remember special moments with friends and the smiles of our beloved family.

When our memory is lacking, it can be frustrating, draining, and confusing. As we age, our memory can become more difficult to manage.

One good thing to know about our memory is that it is unfillable. You will always have room to make more memories. No amount of knowledge is too much for your brain to handle.

The bad news is that the trauma, depression, anxiety, and any other emotional blocks of our vagus nerve can lead to difficulty remembering even the most important things in life.

When we're in the middle of that fight-or-flight response, our brain won't always store the right memories. If you get attacked by a person on the street, you might remember the smell of the mugger, the reflection of the rainwater on the pavement, or the glowing street sign. You might not be as easily remember the color of the eyes of your attacker or the sound of their voice.

Different memories will be created in various situations—no two people will have the same account for what happened, even if they both lived through identical moments.

The vagus nerve is responsible for signaling the brain, so control over these responses will enable you to create better memories.

We often struggle to remember situations because that

fight/flight response was activated. We were struggling to make sense of a situation since we were too busy making sure our defenses were prepared and we were safe from harm.

If you are constantly thinking about the past or worrying over the future, it's impossible to make long and substantial memories of what's around you now.

When the vagus nerve is activated, it helps your brain slow down. You put your mind at ease and tell the rest of the body it's okay to chill. When there is no rushing around in your brain to raise your defenses, you can notice your surroundings—or, should I say, stop and smell the roses.

Memory creation certainly occurs during times of great stress. You dropped an entire bowl of cereal all over your new carpet, and that memory reminds you to carry the bowl with two hands next time. Your purse was stolen from your car and that reminds you to always keep your door locked, even in your driveway.

Memories are useful to us, but too many worried memories can cloud our judgment. If all we ever think about are the bad and terrible things that have happened, it's easy to lose sight of what's good in life and instead focus on all the terror that surrounds us.

The best way to unlock your vagus nerve is through:

- Controlling responses
- Deep breathing
- Meditation
- Healthy environments
- Yoga

The next four chapters are going to lay these essential steps out for you to ensure you are creating a life that maintains a healthy vagus nerve.

CHAPTER 4

THE SOCIAL ASPECT OF THE VAGUS NERVE

The nerve fibers in our vagus system help us to ensure we have proper freeze responses. The regulation of our heart beating, breathing, and all other reactions remind us that we are capable of expressing calm reactions and vocal tones to others.

Whenever we begin to overlook our ability to have civil discussions with the people around us, relationships can become complicated. One person's vagal reactions might be out of balance, and two can mean double the trouble.

It's hard enough to attempt to share messages with other people. Not everyone will understand where we're coming from, and we can struggle internally to come up with the right things to say. Even when we try to get our message across and the other person actively listens, there is a challenge with making sure the point was interpreted properly.

It's easy to see how unhealthy social lives can cause distress. You might be entirely disconnected from society.

Perhaps you struggle to find people you can relate to. It can be very isolating when we're alone with our thoughts.

You are the only one that will ever see the perspective you carry now. Others can try to understand where you're coming from, but there are still many chances for the messages to get lost in transit. The vagus nerve, as we've already discussed, is responsible for sending reactions to the brain. Even within our neurological systems, we can struggle to send the right signals from one part of our body to the next. A lot happens from one person's brain to another, so the more tuned in we are with our neurological functions, the easier it will be not only for others to hear where we're coming from, but for us to know what we mean ourselves.

Those with a higher vagus tone have been determined to have a higher level of connectedness towards others. In general, this makes them experience more frequent positive emotions.

Giving off positivity is a great way to mend relationships. You're ensuring that the other person is not offended by what you have to say and that you are properly spreading important messages. But finding this calm feeling to exude to others is challenging when we aren't checking in with our thoughts and feelings.

When someone might say something aggressive, offensive, or even slightly defensive, it could make someone with an imbalanced vagus nerve struggle to react appropriately. This is where angry outbursts occur and feelings can get hurt.

The vagus nerve can have an impact on social behavior, and as social creatures, we must discover methods of overcoming obstacles in our path to recovery.

Social Interaction

Social interaction is important for a healthy life. We are pack animals. This means we require a tribe-like structure to help us feel fulfilled. Before you could order food to your house through your phone or have security cameras for defense, we lived in a world where we actively depended on other people. Some individuals were stronger physically and able to go out and fight for food. Others were more knowledgeable, staying away from danger while preparing meals or teaching and nurturing others.

What you couldn't do for yourself could be fulfilled by other people.

In a way, that is still biologically required, depending on your goals. If you want to have a home and a family one day, you need other people to start the family. Even if you adopt as a single parent, someone still has to birth the children, and the children are other individuals themselves.

If your goal is to become a famous singer, you need fans, producers, and managers. Even if you don't feel as though you are dependent on others or that you are better off alone, you might be surprised at just how attached you are to your tribal roots. If you woke up tomorrow and you were the last person alive, what would you do? Where would you go? How would you act?

The first few days would be great. You'd be able to snag whatever clothes you want from the mall. You could eat endless snacks from the grocery store. You can get cars and drive anywhere you wanted.

However, after a few weeks, you'd likely get really lonely. You might struggle to understand what your purpose is and you'd long for that deep connection.

We all need moments alone. The overstimulation of all the people that surround us on top of opposing viewpoints and combating personalities can be mentally and physically draining.

We are still wired, as humans, to desire that longing connection with another person, however. We are seeking out that reminder that we are not alone in this, and others feel the same way.

We were given the fight-or-flight responses for a reason. Even though we require social interaction for internal fulfillment, we have also trained our brains to be on the defense. There are a few core fears that we all have. These include:

- Extinction
- Separation
- Mutilation
- Loss of autonomy
- Ego death

If we feel as though any one of these factors is being threatened by another individual, it can signal that fight-or-flight response. This doesn't just occur socially, but situationally as well. For social interactions can cause us to be aggressive toward others or shut them out. If you are getting reprimanded by your boss, you might argue with them defensively, trying desperately to prove your point. You might also completely shut down, sitting there and simply listening as they yell. Any sort of stressor seen in another person can trigger those emotional reactions brought on by signals from the vagus nerve.

Alternatively, we also feel good when we see others. Imagine seeing your mother or father after months without visiting. The look on a baby's face as they laugh can be warming. Waking up and seeing the person you love laying there in the morning might make you feel incredibly good. This releases oxytocin.

There's a balance in two important hormones signaled to release—oxytocin and cortisol. When you are socially interacting with another person, your vagus nerve tells your brain which hormones to release. It's sending signals letting it know if this is a good thing – like seeing a baby laugh – so it can send oxytocin. However, if it's a stressful thing – that same baby crying – this can put your brain on high alert.

Whenever we sense our relationships are being threatened, it can cause us to act out in certain ways. Aside from the balance between the release of cortisol and oxytocin, other hormones can be involved in relationships, such as adrenaline. Perhaps your lover is threatening to leave. They are your entire world and you can't imagine life without them. This tells your vagus nerve you are under a great threat. Your brain might release cortisol and put you into high gear, desperate to do absolutely anything and everything to stop them from leaving.

Love can make people do crazy things, and sometimes that's simply because our brains are telling us to try anything to keep the situation from going bad.

When we are constantly on alert, it becomes difficult to see the joy in social interaction around us. If you are always afraid that your lover will leave, you might stress even in the good moments. If you lack self-esteem and think your friends dislike you, you won't enjoy hanging out with them. If you are fearful that everyone in the world is judging you, it can even be hard to leave the house.

Social Media and Isolation

Using social media can easily make us feel very attacked and isolated. As soon as you get online, there will always be opinions and views that are different from your own. On one hand, you might feel as though you are offended by the things that you see. It's easy to get extremely angry at sensationalized articles that are frequently shared online. However, this can also make us feel very reactionary. When you see something that upsets you or that you disagree with, you can quickly fall into a place where your senses are telling you that you are under attack. You might become defensive to the point that you interact with other people online by frequently getting into arguments.

This is telling your brain to be on high alert all the time when you're online. Another aspect of social media is that people curate their lives through their posts to ensure they always are cast in a positive light. You might see somebody who is always posting about how great their life is, sharing images of their happy family.

It makes you feel isolated. You might not have the things

that others are sharing, so you feel like an outcast from the rest of the world.

A huge part of this is because people aren't posting the negative aspects online. They're only going to be sharing with you the good things in their life. Nobody's going to post about their unpaid bills, a fight they got in with their spouse or the poop that their child smeared all over the wall.

Some people might post certain raw, unedited and realistic content, but for the most part, editing, Photoshop, and curated pictures are consistently used. That can hurt our self-esteem. We might lack confidence, and that can show through the way we interact with others.

Getting online in general, you can constantly find new material. Whether you're watching 10-second videos over and over again, or you're scrolling through a news page and seeing 10 articles in a minute, your brain is always being stimulated. Your senses are always on alert. At any moment you might scroll up and find the one video that makes you upset.

Perhaps you're scrolling through your social media feed and everything is fine until you get to a picture of your girlfriend in a bikini. A few guys are commenting on how great she looks, sending you into a fit of rage and jealousy that makes you lash out at your girlfriend.

Alternatively, maybe you're scrolling through, looking at news articles, and everything seems fine until you get to the one that relates to you.

Our brains have not yet evolved to catch up with this constant stimulation. We go from watching a 10-second video of a puppy running around to reading an article about something horrific like a pedophile ring.

The constant swapping from two dramatically different stimulations is confusing to our senses. Our bodies don't know how to feel or react in these situations. It can be damaging to our perspective and make us feel constantly overstimulated.

The vagus nerve is all about balancing between making

you feel good or making you feel like you are on high alert. If we're not careful, we can disrupt that balance, making it react inappropriately in unrelated situations.

One thing you can do right now is to pay attention to the way that you are using social media.

The Internet is not a bad thing. It can significantly improve our lives for the better. We just have to be careful about how we're using it.

If you go online multiple times a day, only to look at things that upset you like friends you're jealous of or disturbing news articles, then you're not using it for good.

It's good to stay in touch with friends and we always want to be well informed, but you have to remember to establish that balance because your body is going to be reacting in a consistently negative way.

Begin by tracking your social media use. Log how many hours and minutes you're spending in a day.

As you're tracking this time, ask yourself how you're feeling. Rate your mood before you get on and then after you close the app. If your mood is constantly decreasing and you're spending hours a day online, it's time to make some significant changes. If you notice that you only get on maybe 30 minutes here or there, and you feel pretty much the same or even better afterward, then your social media habits are in a healthy place, and that's good to nurture.

Your challenge to better relax your mind and stimulate those important nerves is to begin to unfollow accounts that make you upset.

Challenge yourself to unfollow five people that don't provide you with any good feelings. Even if it's a friend, it's okay to unfollow people online. That doesn't mean you have to cut them out in real life.

Now, go out and find five accounts that make you feel good about yourself. Maybe it's a body positivity account. Perhaps it's one that shows kittens and puppies all the time. Maybe it's an artist who shares their work. Food accounts can make us feel very good too. Use social media as a way to enhance your life and increase your knowledge. Don't use it to provide you with information that isn't necessary and just bring you down. Focus on what's most important, and that's when you'll feel the best.

Body Language

Your vagus nerve correlates with your ability to interpret the body language of others, as well as show signals in your behavior. Social cues are all around us.

These cues come easy to us. Holding the door for the person behind you is polite and expected. Saying thank you after somebody gives you something is common knowledge. Leaving the room when you notice two people are fighting is kind. Asking if somebody is okay after they fall to the ground is anticipated. Social cues occur everywhere and we don't even have to second-guess or think about them twice.

Many of our social cues are automatic and they are a way that we share further information with somebody. But body language is not just using your hands to point, clapping, or other obvious forms of communication. It encompasses everything from the way we furrow our brow to the direction that we're pointing our toes. Without realizing it, we're giving off social cues regularly. Some people might be picking up on these, and letting it negatively affecting a situation.

They might think that you're anxious, therefore they begin feeling anxious, too. These social cues can play off of each other to communicate messages from one body to the next without the mind even understanding all that is going on.

You must begin to notice your body language. The more aware you can be of your body, the easier it will be to begin to interpret that of others.

When we are looking at body language, there are some dangerous cues that you also need to be aware of.

For example, somebody crossing their arms can make you feel closed off and disconnected. Eyes that are jerky and going back and forth around the room might make you feel uneasy or nervous.

Your body is always on alert. It's your vagus nerve's job to ensure that if a threat is suspected, your body is prepared to fight it off. Have you ever walked into a room and instantly felt like you could smell the negative energy or pick up that something was wrong? Nobody said anything, but you were able to recognize a negative situation just by being there.

Your body picked up on the social cues that others are giving, from the way that they are using their limbs, faces, and the rest of their bodies.

If you walk into a room of 10 people and all of them have angry expressions on their faces, that's going to instantly let your body know to be on the defense. These people are mad, and anger shows itself in different ways. Who knows if somebody is going to lash out on you, right? This is all that your body is telling you so that you remain alert.

Pay attention to how you are using every part of your body, from your face to your feet.

The more aware you are of the messages you're trying to express, the simpler it can be to begin to analyze those of others.

How are you placing your hands? What face are you making as somebody else tells you a story? How are your legs situated? Is your posture open or closed off? All of these can be indications of somebody else of the things you're feeling.

Our body expresses these messages without our awareness. Our words can be the way that we filter out these messages. You might be extremely angry, but you are in control of your emotions. You're not letting anybody else know, verbally, that you are upset. However, people that know you well and love you are likely closer to you than others.

They can better recognize the messages you're sending with your body language. They notice that your leg is shaking and that you have an annoyed expression on your face. They're paying attention to the way that you are pacing around the room, upset and angry.

Without your having to express anything out loud, the people around you can pick up on the actual way that you're feeling.

This can be hard to control because your body is sending all these nerves and signals around, telling you how to express yourself to other individuals.

Reading and Showing Body Language

Signals from your vagus nerve to your brain can create facial responses that you may not always be aware of. You could be unknowingly giving other people signals for how they should feel in your presence. You might make someone uncomfortable, making yourself uncomfortable.

To understand how to read your body language and that of others, you have to know what the signs and signals are. Let's start from the top of your head. First and foremost, the direction that your head is turned is going to tell a lot about you. If somebody is sitting next to you on a couch and your face is turned toward them, it shows you're actively listening. If your head is instead turned to face the TV, then it's likely you're more checked out. Eye contact is a huge part of body language.

If you are always looking around, it shows you might not be listening. However, if you stare directly into their eyes the entire time they talk, you could be making them feel uncomfortable. They might be nervous from too much eye contact and you could even be giving them the idea that you're not actually listening, but instead pretending to pay attention.

What we do with our mouth also tells a lot about how

we are feeling or what we may be thinking. If your hand is over your mouth, covering and hiding it from other people, it gives them the idea that you might be keeping something back.

If your lips are curled or sucked in, it could also be that you have something on your mind that you want to say, but your body's telling you to keep it in.

Maybe somebody is telling you a suggestion for a project, but you don't think it's a very smart idea. You don't want to hurt their feelings or maybe it's not even your place to say, so you place your hand over your mouth to keep you from responding.

You might not even be realizing your body is doing this, but it can make you look like you are in deep thought.

Moving down to your arms and shoulders, these will tell the most about what you are thinking or feeling. If your arms are crossed and closed off, it makes you seem like you are not fully listening to the other person or that you are defensive.

If you have your hands on your hips, it might look like you're trying to control the area, using a wide reach in an attempt to gain power over the people around you. Any one of these signs or signals can indicate other individual unspoken messages.

Our legs will also tell a lot about us. The direction that you're pointing your feet might indicate where you want to be. If you're sitting at a party, talking to somebody on the couch, you might have your feet pointed away just because it's a more comfortable position. However, it could indicate that you are interested in talking to the person across the room because that's where your feet are pointed.

Any body-language signs that you're giving off could also be what others are telling through their nonverbal cues.

Every situation is going to be different—somebody might have their arms crossed because they're angry, or they might just have their arms crossed because they're cold.

Body language is not looking at one specific signal and

especially doesn't involve using the exact words somebody states. Pay attention to their eye movement, their tone of voice, how they use their arms and legs, and their body as a whole. They are an entire network of a person, not just one simple signal. You want to have a little background information on them, or at least have a sense of their personality to gain an idea of what behavior is typical.

Some people are extremely expressive with their hands and their face as they speak. Other people won't give you anything at all, so if they did start using their hands, that may indicate to you that they are upset. Look at every aspect of what another individual is trying to tell you and never underestimate the messages that are communicated through their body.

Traumatic Triggers

Any form of trauma is going to skew your ability to socially interact, both verbally and nonverbally. Your body is always going to be wary of experiencing that trauma again. Your vagus nerve sends signals to your brain that it might just endure that same experience when a threat is perceived.

The possible dangers that are sent to your brain aren't always similar. Sometimes they're things that wouldn't bother many, and other times they're situations that call for a greater emotional response. For example, a war veteran might hear a car backfire and, thinking it's a gunshot, cower in fear because they were triggered back to that moment. Alternatively, they might simply see a tree that reminds them of one they saw when in the war, and that causes them to be triggered once again. The signs and signals aren't always the same, and we can't predict everything that will trigger our memory. It involves our vagus nerve telling our brain that we are likely to experience that trauma once again.

If you've experienced great trauma, you might be attuned to look for danger cues even when there are none there. You have unknowingly trained your vagus nerve to respond in a stressful way because of the experiences you endured.

The safer you feel, the easier it will be for you to interact. The best way to ensure that you are feeling safe is to know what your triggers are. This way, you can either avoid them or overcome them.

If you want to overcome your triggers, it begins by decreasing exposure. If you are constantly stimulating yourself, it can be hard to heal. It's like picking at the wound. For example, if your trigger is your mother because she abused you as a child, you will want to cut contact for a while. You might think you can still live with her while you heal, but it can be nearly impossible. It's like trying to cure yourself with the same medicine that made you sick.

You will want to eventually introduce some triggers to overcome them. Not all need to be dealt with, especially in extreme circumstances. For example, if you were mugged in an alleyway, maybe you don't need to walk down alleyways anymore. If you were mugged in a car, however, it might be impossible to avoid cars, so you would want to eventually reintroduce this trigger healthily. It's not an easy process and it requires time and effort to train your vagus nerve to respond appropriately. It's not impossible, either—it starts with knowing what it is that causes a traumatic reaction in your body.

Knowing Triggers

If you know what triggers you, it's easier to understand how it makes you feel. Once you see how you feel in that situation, you're better to be able to know how that is causing your body to react.

For example, you might be triggered by spiders—they make you feel scared, so your body reacts by completely freezing in any situation associated with a spider.

First, try to identify what your trauma might be. It's okay to not have a clear picture, and you might not know all that was involved in those traumatic experiences. Perhaps you were abandoned as a child. It's hard to see all the intrinsic ways this changes our perspective, but upon reflection, you can unearth many symptoms.

Once you know what the basic trauma was, you can begin to notice triggers that are usually associated with the situation. If your trauma was a car accident, cars, car keys, seatbelts, and everything in between might be triggers. These are common traumas:

- Abuse
- Accident
- Harassment
- Torture
- Witnessing violence
- Experiencing violence
- Bullying
- Threats
- Fire
- Starvation/dehydration
- Sexual assault
- Death

Trauma is much more than a singular experience with a few triggers. It can be extremely complex and usually involves elongated periods of extended trauma. These might include things like multiple abusive family members, consistent neglect as a child, poverty, and so on.

When you don't have a specific instance to remember, like a death or an accident, you might not think you have trauma. This isn't always the case. To help you recognize your triggers, you want to look at what feelings they evoke.

For example, maybe you were often made to feel stupid as a child. Every time you asked a question, you were mocked and no one ever helped you with homework. When you go to a party and are chatting with people and someone corrects a fact you stated, it might make you feel like your intelligence is insulted and this triggers you into a freeze reaction.

Your neurology told the rest of your body that you were experiencing trauma once again. It reacted just the way that it did when you were a child, leaving you frozen and helpless.

This emotion isn't an easy one to deal with, but you can start to notice what those triggered feelings are to appropriately respond in that situation. Emotional triggers might make you feel:

- Forgotten
- Neglected
- Cast aside
- Isolated
- Excluded
- Powerlessness
- Out of control
- Disrespected
- Embarrassed
- Humiliated
- Frustrated
- Angry
- Lonely
- Sad
- Hopeless
- Manipulated
- Controlled
- Unsafe
- Unloved

These are just a few of the many different types of triggering emotions. If you notice yourself triggered and feeling one of these kinds of ways, it's important to implement the exercises that we have for you in the next two chapters.

62

CHAPTER 5

NURTURING YOUR VAGUS NERVE

There are practical methods, like deep breathing and yoga, that can help nurture your vagus nerve. Nurturing this nerve, however, extends beyond merely participating in practical exercises. You want to seek ways that you can consistently improve the environment in which your vagus nerve exists. You are deserving of a carefully thought-out lifestyle that ensures your vagus nerve will not be disrupted.

You don't just want to do yoga for 30 minutes a day and not think again about your neurological functions. Maintaining a healthy vagus nerve should be a consistent attempt at enhancing your health. Everything from how you talk to another person to the exercises that you do will send sensory information throughout your body.

Pay special attention to the way that you're feeling to notice any improvements as you enhance your behavior. To begin, check your vagus nerve now. Coughing and gagging are the quickest ways to activate it. Make a note of how you feel before, and then force yourself to cough for 15 to 30 seconds. Don't strain your throat to the point that you feel like you're going to throw up, or that you even scratch it. But give yourself those deep belly coughs, because that can activate it.

Gagging is another way. You might not want to do this if you have a sensitive gag reflex, or you could end up throwing up.

This is when a doctor would take that wooden stick and place it on your tongue to check if your body is functioning properly through your vagus nerve. You can try this on your own, but be very cautious, so that you don't make yourself throw up.

Elongate the health of not just this nerve, but your life. It's important to create a nurturing environment.

A Healthy Environment

When creating a healthy environment, there are four corners to our health that need special attention. Every single part of your body is interlocked. If one part is out of whack, or imbalanced, it can have ripple effects on the rest of your body.

The first corner of your health is nutrition. The things that you eat, or the things that you don't eat, will affect your body. If you are constantly eating junk food and never allow a vegetable into your meals, this will negatively impact your health. If you are constantly eating healthy greens, good protein, and other fruits, that's great! However, you can't overlook the other three corners of your health.

The second is exercise. This is how you're moving your body and what activity you put it through.

The third is your sleep pattern. Are you getting the right amount of rest?

The fourth is your stress level. Are you managing the anxiety or negative emotions that you experience?

If we want to create a healthy environment, we have to place these four pieces of our health together like a puzzle. They connect all that is good and necessary to live a happy and healthy life.

These are all going to affect your vagus nerve. Being hungry all the time, or lacking proper nutrition, tells your body that you need to eat more. Even if you've eaten a lot of junk food in a day, you might not have gotten your proper nutrition, so you could still feel hungry because your body is seeking that out.

If you're too sleepy, that tells your body that you need rest. You might be highly anxious because you are lacking one of these aspects. Maybe you're thirsty, you're stressed, you're hungry and you're tired. This is going to impact the way your body reacts, as an animal.

When any of these areas is lacking, it sends our body into high alert and makes us feel scared and anxious, not knowing what might occur if we aren't careful. You're depriving your body of its basic needs if you are lacking in any of these four corners, so we must ensure we nurture each aspect to keep the vagus nerve functioning properly.

Best Habits

Creating habits is the best way to alter your vagus nerve. There are already wirings and mechanisms within your body that aren't going to change overnight.

Even if you wake up tomorrow a whole new person, ready to implement new habits, that doesn't mean your body is prepared to do the same. Sometimes, it takes a little catching up to get on board with where our mentality is. You want to focus on creating healthy patterns in your life. The more you practice these things, the easier it will be for them to seep into your world. Notice any bad habits that already exist. Do you stay up late and wake up early? Do you stay up late and sleep too late? Do you not eat all day but then binge eat at night? Do you eat throughout the day, but not a healthy amount of food? Pick up on these negative habits and notice the way that they might be affecting your vagus nerve.

If you are constantly tired, then you're not giving yourself the full rest needed. That will keep your body on high defense because if you were to be attacked you wouldn't have the energy to fight the other person off. This is concerning your neurological system, so your body is not going to be able to relax as it should.

Not only will you be tired, but you will be stressed out. Set realistic goals for yourself. It's easy to say that tomorrow you want to wake up and be healthy, but that's not realistic. It's going to take a couple of weeks for you to implement and stick to new habits. The harder you try each day, the easier tomorrow is, but we won't always know exactly how we feel from a day-to-day basis.

Come up with realistic ideas for what you believe you can achieve to set yourself up for success. Pay attention to how you're speaking to yourself. Maybe you do have negative habits—that's not such a bad thing. However, you might tear yourself up for this, or feel bad that you're not good enough.

You're telling your body to be stressed out and scared when you shouldn't be. Focus on relaxation, and make sure that you prioritize time for de-stressing. You are capable of cultivating this life on your own—it's important for your health to do so. Let's go over a few practical exercises that you can begin to implement into your daily life.

Cold Exposure

Cold exposure can help you increase the parasympathetic activity in your body and decreases sympathetic activity. This means that you help your breathing regulate, while the stress response is properly managed.

Too much cold can be harmful, so you must allow yourself to do this only in small bursts.

Cold exposure sounds just as you think it would. It's exposing your body to cold sensations. This kicks that vagus nerve into high alert, but the instant release of warm afterward reminds your body that you are safe and protected. Not only does this naturally occur in your body, but you are also training yourself to be calm in a stressful situation.

Exposing your body to extreme cold can make it freak out. Being too cold can be harmful, so your body is going to want to avoid this to protect yourself. If you put yourself in this naturally dangerous situation with a positive and relaxed mindset, you are making it easier for your brain to be relaxed later on. To begin with, cold exposure starts by simply using ice cubes. Have ice-cold water, or sip on a cool drink. Eat a popsicle.

Doing this can be simple enough to help relax you and keep you focused at the moment. Then, take it to a more intense level. Take a cold shower. You don't even have to jump in the shower right when it's cold. Maybe you step in when it's warm and gradually decrease the temperature. Alternatively, you can jump into a cold shower, but then eventually increase the temperature until it's warm.

Give your body small bursts of cold, because that can help kickstart the important functions of your vagus nerve. You can simply stick your head in the freezer for a moment, or step outside into the snow. More extreme versions of cold therapy include ice baths. Sometimes, people will fill up their tub with cold water and ice. They will submerge themselves just for a few seconds, and then come out. Not only is this giving your body a blast of cold, but you're also challenging your mind to stay calm and relaxed. You're testing your brain and realizing just how much power you have over the thoughts and actions that you experience.

Targeted Massages

Massaging the body anywhere is important for circulation and the release of tense and sore muscles. If you can get a professional massage, absolutely do this.

Massaging your body isn't just a one-time spot treatment. We should be considering it as a consistent therapy for our bodies. We often don't realize how we hold tension, and even the way that we frequently sit can be terrible for our posture.

Massage is a gradual process. Your body won't get back to where it should be after one session. You should consistently work through these kinks to eventually have a healthier body. When it comes to your vagus nerve, you can begin to massage yourself in targeted areas to stimulate those senses.

Pay attention to your neck. Place your hand on the area where your neck meets your shoulder. Start with two fingertips and slowly work your way up toward your ear lobes. Go back around your neck. Don't press too hard to the point that it hurts; it should be a good feeling.

Move your hands upwards in consistent motion and you will discover this is a great way to help begin to release some tension.

Your foot is also an important area for targeted massages. Hold your foot and place your thumb right below your toes. Move down to the center of your foot. Press there and continue to move your thumb up and down in the same motion. Doing this stimulates your vagus nerve and helps get your blood flowing.

Physical Balance

Thirty minutes of movement every day is all that is recommended. It doesn't matter if you get 30 minutes of running in or just dance for half an hour. Whatever you do, try to get an average of 30 minutes of activity each day. This means you could also get two hours one day, and one hour the next, with a few fifteen-minute exercises here and there. This must end up just being the average.

Focus on cardio and repetition. This is going to be best for stimulating your vagus nerve. Light exercises help release tension and make you feel more focused and driven. Anything too strenuous might stress you out or cause unwanted tension and sore muscles throughout your body. It's not that this is a bad thing for you in general, but when it comes to stimulating your vagus nerve, focus on the reduction of stress first.

Stay hydrated through your workouts. Always drink plenty of water before you start for energy and replenish your hydration afterward if you sweat a lot throughout the workout.

Nutritional Vagal Practices

Balancing your diet can increase the health of your vagus nerve. The food you eat is one of the four corners of your health, so focus on eating the right things.

One sneaky thing that might affect your vagus nerve is how much sugar you are taking in. Sugar comes from sweet things like candy and baked goods. However, it's also hidden in plenty of our savory foods, like white bread, pasta, salad dressing, yogurt, and much more.

Too much sugar can constantly activate your brain. It will keep you on high alert and feeling more stressed out than you need to be. By reducing your sugar and caffeine intake, you can better relax your body.

Probiotics

There are 100 billion neurons in your brain, but 500 million in your gut. It wouldn't be a completely false statement to say our stomachs do have a mind of their own! When it comes to balancing your nutrition, you must repair any damage done to your stomach with probiotics.

Our stomach is a microbiome, which means there are trillions of bacteria in our stomachs, all living to keep our health balanced. When we don't eat right, we can damage those bacteria. Eating isn't the only thing that will do this—

too much and frequent stress can also begin to destroy our microbiome. Probiotics will help to repair those living things essential for proper digestion.

Probiotics can help to reduce that stress. They ensure that we are maintaining a higher level of health and feeling good more frequently. Probiotics can be taken in supplement form. Prebiotics can also be used to help feed your stomach so that you can create healthy probiotics. Many capsules and supplements will contain both or at least have a suggested pairing.

Other than supplements, you can include these probiotic foods in your diet for greater health:

- Yogurt (Greek is usually best, stay away from artificial sweeteners)
- Kefir
- Cottage cheese
- Sauerkraut
- Kimchi
- Kombucha

Any fermented food is going to help maintain your microbiome. Ensure you are choosing fermented foods, which take a while to change form through the use of alcohol, and not pickled, which is a flavor changer with salt and vinegar.

Omega-3s

DHA is essential for your brain health. It:

- Increases plasticity
- Reduces stress
- Regulates oxygen
- Promotes learning
- Increases memory

DHA is mostly found in omega-3 fatty acids, which can be taken as supplements to ensure proper stimulation of the vagus nerve. You can also find many different foods that contain these essential fatty acids, such as:

- Salmon
- Tuna
- Mackerel
- Sardines
- Oysters
- Anchovies
- Cod
- Seaweed
- Shrimp
- Hemp seeds
- Chia seeds
- Flaxseeds
- Avocado
- Kidney beans
- Walnuts

72

Are you enjoying this book? I'd like to know what you think, leave me a short review on Amazon, thanks again!

CHAPTER 6

BREATHING AND MEDITATION

Your vagus nerve is responsible sensations experienced through the lungs, the stomach, and the heart. These are all very important parts of your body and all share that they are regulated with your breathing. Your lungs filter the air in and out of your body daily without you having to think about it. When you're zoned out watching TV, working hard at your computer, or passed out in bed, your lungs are still working constantly. You can stop your lungs, but eventually, that feeling automatically kicks in for you to begin to breathe again.

You need to breathe to provide air to every aspect of your body.

When we cut off circulation, that part can become permanently damaged. We don't realize just how irregular our breathing patterns can be. Sometimes, though you might breathe in and out, and you're not getting the full amount of air required to help you feel better.

Using breathing and meditation has a plethora of health benefits that enable you to relax and calm your body. You can stimulate your vagus nerve through deep breathing. You're lowering your heart rate, you're regulating your breath, and you're calming your stomach. Your mind is at peace because you are focused on one thing at a time.

There are so many things happening in the world at any given moment, it can be hard to catch our breath. By focusing on deep breathing, you show your vagus nerve that you are safe and protected. It can remind the rest of your body that being on an extreme level is unnecessary.

Breathing and meditation help with depression management, too. Sometimes, we don't realize just how panicked we are. You might be in a depressive state where you can't get out of bed. Even though it seems like you are being calm, internally, you might be experiencing so much anxiety that your body has chosen to use that freeze response.

You're not moving. You're not going anywhere, and you have no desire to do anything because you are so overwhelmed and stressed.

To people on the outside, you might just seem like somebody lazy laying in bed. Anybody with depression knows that internally, it is a constant struggle. There is nothing fun or easy about suffering from constant depressive moods.

These mood swings can negatively affect every area of our life. Of course, regulating your breath does not cure major depression. However, focusing on your breathing can begin to alleviate some of the symptoms brought on by depression. You're not going to turn your life around, and breathing one time for five minutes isn't going to cure you of your past traumas. But breathing can stop you from a panic attack.

If you notice that your heart is racing and your mind is going a million miles per minute, you can start to counteract that by breathing. Focus on your counting, feel the air coming into your body, and notice the way you feel as it leaves. This can calm you more than you could know.

To boost your energy, you can use breathing exercises. If you're feeling unmotivated or unfocused, you can take 10 minutes away and give your brain that oxygen.

This lets your vagus nerve know you are protected at this moment and nothing is going to harm you.

Self-Control and Discipline

Vagal breathing helps teach us proper self-control and discipline.

It's easy to notice your anxious thoughts and recognize when you're experiencing these situations, but it's not as simple to know how to stop them.

It requires a lot of emotional discipline to step back from rumination or brooding and say, "Okay, this isn't helpful, I need to refocus." Nobody wants to have anxious thoughts, even when they recognize that they need to go away.

Your self-control and discipline can drastically increase as you are practicing mindfulness meditation and breathing exercises. You're regaining power over your stimulation. You're noticing your senses and reminding yourself that you are in a relaxed and safe space. You are calm and you are protected, and nothing is going to hurt you. When you are focused on your breathing, you recognize that even if you do experience some pain, it will be so deeply felt because you are in control of your emotions. When somebody makes you upset, rather than lashing out and freaking out back at them, you can control your response and decide to have a healthy discussion with this person.

You can come to a conclusion, make agreements, and find compromise when at least one person in the situation is remaining emotionally calm. Deep breathing helps you gather your thoughts to respond in a way that is beneficial to all parties involved.

Self-control is important because we want to be the ones in charge of how we respond neurologically to a situation. Self-control allows you to hone in on your emotional reaction.

When a situation is causing you extreme distress, rather than feeling panicked and on the defense, you can ensure that you approach the situation calmly. You can focus on doing what is most important and pay attention to the task at hand.

Rather than dwelling on the anxious thoughts that consume your brain power, you're telling your senses you have the solution, and you are in control of the situation.

Breathing is the only way that we will be able to make ourselves feel better, even when the reality of the worst-case scenario has come true. When our deepest, darkest prophecies are fulfilled, we can still make it through the situation if we just focus on breathing.

Mindfulness

Mindfulness is the act of being aware of your surroundings. When we are feeling anxious and stressed, that tells our vagus nerve to kick into high gear.

That balance between feeling relaxed and prepared becomes strained. If you are never present in the moment and always thinking of the past or looking towards the future, you are trapped in an endless mental cycle. You're not giving your brain that chance to calm down and relax.

This can mean being on the defensive all the time. You might be ready and prepared to yell at anybody who tests your ego. You might snap at the next person who says something slightly wrong. You might be constantly afraid, always ready for the worst thing to happen. You're prepared for the absolute worst possible outcome.

This will keep you mentally exhausted. You want to allow yourself to feel good and calm. It's great to be prepared, but always getting stuck in a place where you are stressed is using the power of your vagus nerve in the wrong way.

Mindfulness pulls your anxious thoughts of the future

and your regret or guilt over the past and brings your focus to what is going on around you. There are a few simple mindfulness activities you can incorporate into your daily life.

Do these as you do the breathing techniques for optimum focus in the next section.

The first act of mindfulness is to simply think of a color. The first color that comes to your mind is fine, but pick something basic like green, blue, purple, red, and so on. Avoid anything too obscure, like chartreuse or periwinkle.

Think of the first color and identify everything in the space you are currently in that is that color. Maybe you're sitting in the park. Perhaps you're behind your desk at work. Maybe you're riding the train home. Look around you and find everything that is this specific color. If your color is green, notice the green leaves on the trees. Notice the green pencil holder on your desk. Pay attention to the green cars you pass on the train. This is a simple way to be mindful.

You're pulling the focus from wherever you were in your brain and turning it toward everything that surrounds you. Another act of mindfulness is to tap into your five senses. Notice one thing you can smell, one thing you can see, one thing you can touch, one thing you can hear, and one thing you can taste. You don't have to taste or smell these items, but pick them out.

Again, if you're at the park, you smell the leaves, you could taste the ice cream that somebody is eating across from you. When you're on the train, you feel the lurch as the train goes over a bump. Sitting behind your desk, you hear your coworker talking about her dog. Be mindful at the moment by noticing your surroundings, which makes your thoughts easier to control. This alleviates pressure on your vagus nerve and reminds your body that you are calm and protected.

Beginner Exercises

Everyone already knows how to breathe. We are all fully capable of inhaling and exhaling. However, we don't realize all of the power that we have with each of these breaths. Some people will be able to breathe so deeply they feel a rush in their mind, almost a high.

If you feel light-headed during any of these activities, make sure to give yourself breaks in between. A little lightheadedness isn't terrible—you will notice that the rush helps to relax your body. Don't do anything too quickly, as deep rapid breathing can stress you out. Make sure your breaths are slow and that you are not depriving your body of the air that it needs.

You can do these exercises anytime, anywhere, and as often as needed. Allow yourself to feel your lungs expand as you fill them with air and notice the increase in your stimulation senses afterward.

1 Minute

The first breathing exercise we have for you is rather simple. You can do this whenever you are feeling stressed out. It's a good way to pull in good feelings and blow out any negativity that is weighing on you.

Begin by sitting somewhere comfortable and make sure that your airway is not restricted. Don't lay to where your neck or your chin is cramped, making it harder for you to breathe. Give yourself as much space as possible around you, as well. Don't pile onto your bed with a million pillows and blankets just yet. Spread out and give yourself freedom. For this exercise, you're going to begin by breathing in only through your nose. Close your mouth and inhale as you count to five. Breathe in now for one, two, three, four, and five. Hold it for one second, then breathe out all in one second through your nose.

If you have any issues with your sinuses, you might need a tissue for the first few times you do this. Only do it once every 30 seconds. If you do it too frequently, you're going to stimulate the vagus nerve instead of relaxing it.

Try this again. Breathe in through your nose for five and out through your nose for one. You won't be able to get all of the air out in one, but you do want to try to get it out as quickly as possible. It's a good way to slowly build and then decrease fast.

It's almost like you are an angry bull.

Do this when you are extremely frustrated. If you can feel your fists curling up and your blood boiling, allow yourself to breathe this way. It can immediately alleviate all of your senses. Again, don't do it too frequently or it can cause you to breathe even faster and feel more anxious. Do it a few times in a couple of minutes, then give yourself a break. You can move on to the other breathing exercises once you've calmed down, as well. Remember not to overexert yourself, because then it becomes like an exercise where you might be straining your neurological system.

5 Minute

For this five-minute breathing exercise, you want to sit somewhere comfortably. Let your torso be stretched out and place your hand on your stomach.

Close your eyes and let yourself feel completely relaxed from the top of your head to the bottom of your feet. Again, you're going to breathe in through your nose, but for this exercise, you're going to breathe out through your mouth.

You're going to want to breathe out extremely gently and slowly. Breathe in through your nose as you count to 10. Start at one and count up. Then, as you breathe out, only do so through your mouth in a tiny hole while you count down from 10.

Start from 10 and descend. It will look like this:

Breathe in for one, two, three, four, five, six, seven, eight, nine, and ten. Breathe out for ten, nine, eight, seven, six, five, four, three, two, and one.

If you can't make it to ten, that's fine—do as much as

you can and try to gradually increase.

Keep your hand on your stomach and place your other hand on your chest. If you are right-handed, place your right hand on your stomach. If you are left-handed, place your left hand on the stomach. The other hand goes on your heart.

As you breathe in, feel as your stomach expands. As you breathe out, feel it decrease.

This breathing exercise is perfect if you are having a panic attack. If you feel anxiety overwhelming you, or you're having a fit of rage, stress, or panic, remove yourself from the situation. Place yourself in a new setting and give your body the chance to breathe.

Breathe in again through your nose and out through your mouth. You are concentrating the air and redirecting the focus. Do this for five minutes at the most and then give yourself another break. If you do it too frequently, you might feel dizzy or light-headed.

Breathe in and out, in and out. You are connecting your chest, your stomach, and your breathing. In doing this, you will be able to stimulate your vagus nerve. Remember to not just do these breathing exercises when you are stressed, either.

They are perfect at all moments of the day, whether you are feeling overwhelmed or you need a burst of energy. They're perfect for waking up in the morning and also winding down at night. Sometimes, in the morning, we feel so rushed that it starts our day off terribly. How many times have you felt overwhelmed by waking up just five minutes late? Give yourself a moment to separate from time and space and focus only on your body.

Activate your vagus powers so throughout the rest of the day, you remain calm and collected in any situation you need. Breathe in and out, in and out. Never forget that it will always help you.

15 Minutes

This last 15-minute exercise is a bit longer and almost like a meditation. It is an act of mindfulness, as well. This is what many people refer to as a body scan. You will want to lay perfectly flat and relaxed.

Don't have any of your limbs bent and make sure that you are in a peaceful setting. Give yourself the chance to drift away to sleep, if you have to. Don't do this while you are driving, and make sure that you are not operating anything else dangerous as you begin this breathing exercise.

To begin, you're going to want to continue breathing in through your nose and out through your mouth, like we had you do in the last exercise. Close your eyes and picture nothing but black. Your vision is dark, and you don't see anything around you. Feel the way that the tension releases itself from your head. Breathe in through your nose and out through your mouth.

As you notice your head, think of all the amazing powers that lie beneath your skull—you can see, think, and hear, all within your mind. Your head is one of the most powerful parts of your body. Breathe in and out as you remember this. Move down now to your neck and your shoulders. Breathe in and out as you feel the tension release itself from here.

You often feel like you are carrying the weight of the world on your shoulders, but that is not true. Other people do respect your abilities and you have great power and influence. You do not have to feel the pressure weighing down on these parts of your body.

Breathe in and out as you release this tension. Feel your chest. This is where it hurts the most during heartbreak and feels the best when you are in love. Feel as your heart continues to be so powerful. You don't even have to think about it—this incredible organ does it all on its own.

Breathe in and out as you acknowledge your chest, then move down to your stomach. Notice the way that it expands and decreases as you breathe in and out. Your lungs sit above this, but you feel it most here. That gut feeling also tells you when something is good or bad.

Feel your arms and your legs now. They help carry you. They protect you and give you the power to push through all of these other parts of life.

Breathe in and out, in and out. You might be able to do this in less than 15 minutes, or it might take you longer. Give yourself time to focus on yourself. Breathe in as you think about each part of your body and breathe out as you release the tension. The point of this breathing exercise is to simply keep you grounded at the moment.

Meditation Sessions

Meditation is one of the best ways for you to find the peace needed to calm your vagus nerve.

To meditate, you want to think of nothing at all. You want to completely clear your mind so that nothing distracts you. You might have constant distractions that fill your day, but the intent here is to separate these feelings and instead focus on completely blanking out your thoughts.

Only when you do this can you hit your reset button and find that mental energy needed to conquer the day. To meditate, make sure you pick out a specific location. This goes the same for yoga.

Whether you are meditating or participating in a yoga session, find an exclusive space you can dedicate to this. It should be a space where nothing else happens. It doesn't have to be an entire room, just a section. For example, if you have a small apartment, pick the place next to your bed on the floor. You likely don't do anything here other than walk around, so you can use this space to meditate or do yoga. You just want a completely brand-new perspective to offer you the insight needed for complete and total relaxation.

Aside from this, you also want to make sure that you begin in small amounts. Don't expect that you'll be able to do 30 minutes on the first day. You might only be able to make it up to 15 minutes, or even just five minutes before your brain starts swirling with anxiety once again.

In the next section, we will provide a guided meditation for you to use. Of course, you can do this at your own pace. It might only take you 10 minutes, or you might want to extend it to an entire hour. Set a timer to help you get a sense of how long you are taking. Begin by timing yourself for 10 minutes and then move it to 20, then 30, then 40, then to an hour. Eventually, you'll be able to have hour-long meditation sessions that can reset your vagus nerve. Until you're able to do this, practice in small amounts and use guided meditation as needed. Focus on your breathing and remember that breathing in through your nose and out through your mouth is going to be the best.

30-Minute Guided Meditation

You are completely at ease. Your mind is not thinking anything worrisome at this moment. You are perfectly content with your surroundings. Stretch your arms and legs out now and fold your hands across your stomach if you don't want to keep them next to your sides.

Feel all the tension leaves your body. Close your eyes and focus on nothing. As soon as one thought begins to come into your mind, gently push it away.

Feel yourself fill with air.

Let the air leave your body. Breathe in for 10, and out for 10. Breathe in for 10, and out for 10.

Notice the way that your heart continues to beat as you breathe. Your heartbeat matches that same rhythmic pattern. Breathe in for 10 and out for 10. Imagine that you are in a safe and calm space. Maybe you were sitting along the edge of a grassy plain. Maybe you found the perfect cozy spot to sit on a mountain hike.

Perhaps you have your toes dipped into the water at the beach. Maybe you're simply laying out in the sand, staring up at the sky.

Pick this place now, and feel as the air surrounds you. Breathe in for 10, and out for 10. Breathe in through your nose and out through your mouth. Focus the air. Let thoughts continue to pass through. Each time something comes to your brain, there's no need to force it out. There's no need to confront it, and you don't have to fix the issues that present themselves in your mind.

Imagine that you are in a body of water. A few leaves are falling from a tree above you. Instead of letting the leaves come toward you and stick to your body, you gently guide them away. You don't pick the leaves up and throw them. You don't tear the leaves apart. You don't try to put them back on to the tree. You don't push them under the water. You simply push your hand out and guide the water so that they drift away from you.

Watch as the leaves continue to flow by. You don't need to give in to these leaves. You don't need to give in to these thoughts. Breathe in for ten and out for 10. Breathe in for 10, and out for ten.

Imagine that you are in a grassy pasture. You are safe and protected, sitting on a cozy bench behind a fence. You notice there's a herd of wild horses. These horses are your thoughts. You can either go up to them and try to ride one, no matter how wild and might be, or you can simply enjoy them as they pass. You're not thinking about where they came from or where they're going.

You are only appreciating watching them run, the sounds of their hooves beating on the ground relaxing you. It's like a heartbeat, and the breeze blows through your hair. Breathe in for 10 and out for 10. In for 10 and out for 10. Your mind is empty and blank. Your thoughts are clear, and your focus is connected.

Your body is one, your mind is one, your spirit is one. Together, these are a whole entity that creates the person you are. You are incredibly happy to be alive, you are excited for the day. You know everything that is required to succeed. You are fulfilled, you are thrilled, you are excited. You are relaxed and at peace. Nothing around you disturbs you.

Nothing around you scares you. Everything is good and calm and relaxed and at peace. Breathe in for 10 and out for 10. In for 10 and out for 10.

Let yourself continue to breathe as your mind goes blank. Focus on gently pushing these thoughts away and remember to relax. Center yourself and feel as your vagus nerve becomes at peace.

CHAPTER 7

YOGA

Exercise is always about being fast, pushing yourself, and building muscle. This is great, but sometimes our bodies need to maintain a level of calm in those processes. Yoga is a great exercise to help your body and your mental balance. It is combining practicality with the reduction of your trauma.

Yoga is an ancient practice but has gained popularity in Western culture. You have probably seen many trends like hot yoga, goat yoga, and even people who drink wine during their sessions.

You don't need a fancy studio or a trendy idea to do yoga, though. You can begin by doing so in the morning when you wake up, or in those quick moments before you pop in the shower! Yoga is a great way to reduce the stress that leaves you feeling better about yourself. It stimulates the vagus nerve and activates our senses.

Don't push yourself too far as you begin yoga. Just like any exercise, you will want those warm-up and cool-down phases.

The Yoga-Vagal Connection

Yoga is good for stimulating all parts of your body. However, it is particularly good at activating your heart, lungs, and stomach. When these are relaxed, that will carry signals through your vagus nerve, letting your brain know you are safe and protected. Your vagus nerve is on high alert at all times of the day. It is what catches you when you feel like you're falling, the gut-punch feeling you have when you know something isn't right, and the tingly feeling on your shoulders when you feel like you're being watched.

Much more is involved in the processes that cause these reactions to arise, but it is the Vagus nerve that is responsible for signaling the rest of your body to gear up.

Yoga is all about finding balance. You are required to stay calm and focus on your body and breathing. The kind of slow, deep breathing that yoga requires can induce the same effects that military participants or law enforcement members have to practice when training to deescalate a situation.

The two are connected because yoga is all about creating that balance between your parasympathetic and sympathetic nervous systems. You are reducing your cortisol, telling your brain that everything is going to be okay. You aren't just *relaxing*, but specifically <u>training your brain to be relaxed.</u>

Much of the discomfort is a frame of mind. While physical pain is real, emotional pain can be inflated by our thoughts. Physical pain can also feel worse when we're not properly managing our emotions. You might stub your toe, causing shocking pain in your foot. You can deeply breathe and calm down from this, or you can lash out and throw whatever you're holding across the room. The pain felt might be the same, but the reaction afterward is based on our emotional control.

Sometimes, yoga is uncomfortable at first. You might be forced to deal with the effects of having to stretch a muscle that doesn't normally move in a certain way. Perhaps you're uncomfortable with your body and a yoga class puts you at center stage in front of others who are exercising in similar ways.

You are training your body to embrace what is uncomfortable. Our vagus nerve can sometimes tell our brain to react more than necessary. If you start to breathe fast because you are upset at what your friend is telling you, maybe that sends signals throughout your nervous system that you are under attack. There is a threat and you need to overcome it. You can become defensive and lash out at them.

Your vagus nerve can also tell your body that you are perfectly fine. Everything around you is okay, and even though there is a confrontational moment happening, remaining calm is the way to go.

Yoga gives our bodies a chance to breathe and train our minds so that we can stay strong and focused in all times of discomfort.

Nerve Stimulation

Yoga's greatest asset is that it helps to balance the body. You can rest assured knowing you likely won't have to struggle with a neurological issue when you are consistently practicing yoga. As we mentioned in the first section of this chapter, exercise is often about being quick. That can overstimulate our nerves, confuse our bodies, and cause unnecessary stress. It can also lead to mental exhaustion.

You can be someone who eats healthy all day long, always exercises, and never smokes, drinks, or does anything else negative for their health. If you aren't giving yourself time to relax and balance your vagus nerve, though, you are going to be feeling the negative side effects in the most surprising ways. You might struggle to know what's wrong when you're seemingly doing everything right, but the vagus nerve will have more obvious effects than you'll be able to recognize.

Yoga means flexibility and spreading your powers across your body. You can center yourself and rebalance your energies healthily and positively. It gives you the chance to collect erratic emotions and put them all in a balanced position. You don't have to worry about overstimulating your nervous system when doing yoga because the very intention is to center and calm you.

It promotes posture and balance. You will be more aware of how you are holding your body. Sometimes, we carry tension in our shoulders and arms, not realizing how much strain and stress are being put on our bodies.

It gets your body moving, meaning that the regulation of blood and hormones throughout your body is going to be kept in check. Any exercise is good for that, and yoga is no exception when it comes to the way it induces your breathing and regulates your muscles.

Exercise is something you have to focus on. Regardless of what it does for your mind, it creates the internal ability to stay focused and dedicated to something. You have to carve out a period to do it on a daily or weekly basis. It's required that you warm up, track progress, cool down, and have a relaxation period. Any task that separates your mind from something stressful and puts it toward something more productive is beneficial to your overall health.

Guided Yoga

We have a few guided yoga movements you can do to help you find peace and serenity. Yoga is going to activate your nerves and stimulate your senses. Focus on the beginner moves and your breathing strategies as you attempt the thirty-minute yoga exercise. Again, just like meditation, you will be doing this on your own after the reading so you can either try to shorten it or extend it as you need. Let yourself remain calm and remember this is supposed to relax your mind and put your vagus nerve at ease, not do the opposite.

Beginner Movements

Make sure that you are in a peaceful place to begin these yoga movements. Sit on the ground, preferably with a yoga mat beneath you. If not, simply ensure that you will not be slipping around on the floor as you move. Sit up straight with your legs in front of you and your arms by your sides. Pull your legs into a bent position so the bottoms of your feet are touching. Try to pull your heels as close to your pelvic region as possible. Don't strain yourself, but keep your feet centered. Bring your arms in front of you into a praying position, where your palms are also placed together. Breathe in and out as you hold this pose.

This is one of the best places to start any of your yoga exercises. You can give your body a chance to decompress as you begin to put a great emphasis on your breathing patterns.

Feel the air coming out of your body and a good, fresh air enter. You are centering yourself and this alone is going to begin activating your vagus nerve.

If you want to begin in a standing position, place your feet shoulder-width apart with your hands behind you. Bring your hands together in a praying position once again and lift them toward your chest. Take your right leg and place the bottom of your foot on your left leg, above your left knee. This is what is known as a tree position. Both of these two poses are great starting positions for yoga movements. You'll be able to breathe in and out effortlessly and it makes your vagus nerve stimulated from the moment that you begin.

This is important to know because you want to release the tension and stretch before you start straining your body with other movements.

Next, we're going to teach you the basic breathing methods that will help you get into the right place to do the guided yoga session.

Yoga Breathing

Yoga breathing is all about building.

To notice your breath, grab a mirror or a piece of glass and hold it in front of you. You can simply use a glass cup or stand in front of your bathroom mirror. Blow out through your mouth to fog-up this glass.

Now try to do the same with your nose. What you'll notice is that your breathing is deeper and slower to get the hot steam to fog up the glass.

This is what you want to try to elicit when you are doing yoga breaths. Try to find those deep breathing techniques, because this is going to be the most powerful.

Another yoga breathing move you can try is to make a fist with your right hand.

Stick out your thumb and pinky. Take your right pinky and place it on your left nostril.

Close this nostril and breathe in through your right nostril.

Take your right thumb and place that now on your right nostril, lift your right pinky off of your left nostril and exhale.

Continue this pattern of alternating pinky and thumb, left and right nostrils, to help regulate your breathing. It is a great way to keep your focus centered while you move through this next guided session.

Polyvagal Yoga Session (30 Minutes)

For this yoga session, you are going to start in the sitting position that we discussed with the beginner movements. In the final position, you will be standing in that tree position.

We are going to have you move from one to the next in phases. Focus on your breathing each time. The point of this exercise is to activate your vagus nerve. You're going to calm it down so that it relaxes your mind and your body. You are going to be centered the entire time, focusing on both the left and right parts of your body.

Sit in this position now, with the bottoms of your feet clasped together. Hold your hands in a praying motion and breathe in and out.

Breathe in through your nose and out through your mouth. If you are not yet calm enough to begin, refer back to one of the breathing exercises that we presented in the last chapter, or try using the glass trick to pull those deep breaths from you.

From your position now, bring your arms straight forward in front of you. Reach as far forward as you can and place them on the ground. As slowly and gently as you can, pull your legs out from under you and put yourself into a kneeling position in one movement. Take your time to get here so that you aren't straining any muscles. Slowly now, bring your pelvis to the ground. You will feel the tension leave your body.

Keep yourself flat against the ground from the waist down and push yourself up high with your arms. Your torso will be upwards, with your legs flat on the ground. Push yourself back a little to feel your back stretching. Slowly lift your head and look to the sky. Feel yourself in this position as you breathe in through your nose and out through your mouth.

All in one movement now, bring your behind back up into the air and fold yourself down so that you are on your knees.

Put your head down to the ground and hold this position. Breathe in for 10 and out for 10. Now, raise your behind as high as you can—both your legs are straight and your torso is straight, each at a perpendicular angle to one another. Your hands and feet are both on the ground in what is referred to as a downward-facing dog. Breathe in for 10 and out for 10.

Now you are going to slowly lift yourself using your arms.

You are now in a full standing position. Step forward with your right leg, your right knee bent and pointing out, with your left leg still in place behind you at an angle. Bring your arms out so that one arm is in front of you and the other is behind you. This is what is known as a warrior position.

Breathe in for 10 and out for 10.

Move back to a standing position, and then swap your leg and your arm positions. Hold this once again. Breathe in for 10 and out for 10. Now move back to a standing position.

Bring the bottom of your foot up to your thigh, above your knee in the tree position we mentioned earlier. Breathe in for 10 and out for 10. Bring your leg down now and rest. Repeat one more time for full activation. Challenge yourself to do this movement backward, as well.

You have completed this cycle of meditation, which should take from 10 to 15 minutes. If you are doing it slowly and peacefully, each movement should last a few minutes as you hold it there. Of course, we only told you to breathe in for 10 and out for 10, but do a few rounds of this for each position.

Each time, to fully feel your body relax, you should stay connected and focused and repeat these movements as necessary. This is intended for beginners, so as you continue to stretch and practice, you will become more advanced with what your body can do.

CONCLUSION

To affect change in one's body, we have to know how to send it the right message—and once we know how to send that message, we need to also understand how these messages work and what the outcome will be. Overstimulation is a danger faced by anyone, but it can be exceptionally devastating if you push your own body into this state. Care should be taken at any time when dealing with the body, especially in areas you are yet unfamiliar with.

Many courses of guided meditation and other similar techniques have shown to have boosting effects on the state of one's body, most often toward health. Meditation and breathing exercises, alongside the stress relief of yoga, have affected numerous changes in those suffering from anxiety, depression, and physical pain through triggering the right systems in the body—one of those being the vagus nerve. Not every breathing pattern or yogic positioning can trigger the vagus; in fact, certain patterns and positions will excite the body.

The human body is powerful, and what is key to your health and welfare is understanding how to provide for what it needs. When dealing with pain and trauma, it is best to come to an understanding of the affected area; how it works and how damage to that area will appear, in addition to a course of action to treat this particular damage. Without this information, you're swinging to hit your target, but it's pitch-black and you have no idea what you're swinging for and so each swing could be a mere hairsbreadth away from what you need to do, but it could have no effect at all or produce the exact opposite effect than that of which you desired.

That's why this title is here—to shed some light on what can be a dark matter and to equip you with the specific tools that will be a crutch and an aid in your future. Hopefully, through vigilance and utilizing the exercises within these pages, you will find a balance that has so far been missing from your life.

One such aspect that you may experience could be that you find yourself socially inept, or improperly prepared for general social interaction. This could be due to many things, but one, in particular, is the vagus nerve and its role in both presenting and understanding body language—a crucial part of communication. As social creatures, there is a necessity to overcome any obstruction that is in the path of establishing a healthy social connection. The heavy traffic of communication is further reinforced by the messages that fire through your body, telling you what you're experiencing and allowing you to determine how to react, and then sending those messages to affect that change. If this system breaks down, it becomes difficult to understand and respond.

Coming toward the close of this title, you will find several detailed practical exercises, including the theory and history behind how and why these practices are effective. Part of this is the polyvagal theory, a line of thought that has led to therapeutic recovery through holistic means and has been shown to greatly impact the injured person in these cases. Aspects of this include stimulating the vagus nerves through physical exertion, such as controlled breathing, meditation, and even chanting and yoga. These exercises naturally de-stress and relieve the body while stimulating the nerves without external, man-made aid.

The reasoning and understanding behind our knowledge of the vagus nerve are simply limited to the extent of what we as a race have been able to study and identify, and so not everything about the vagus nerve has been uncovered. As of yet, the new understanding recent studies have shown are creating burgeoning fields within the medical and psychiatric disciplines—even to the extent of creating new divisions of study within these areas of expertise.

While these have been great leaps for mankind, they are not all necessarily implicating the individual directly, but perhaps peripherally by expanding potential career opportunities.

There are much freedom and confidence to be gained through these practices. You are the one who is the most in charge of these emotions, and we have to recognize this great strength. Nobody else is going to provide us with the power to take care of ourselves—this ability lies within our own hands. Remind yourself regularly to check in with your vagus nerve. If you are feeling lethargic, upset, or anxious, ask yourself, "Have I taken care of my senses today? Am I overstimulated?"

It can be easy to have a headache and assume the worst. Even if you don't have any symptoms, you might still panic that you're one of the rare cases that you only see on the news. Perhaps you have a rare disease that no one else has ever had before. They'll name it after you because it's so rare!

These anxious thoughts disrupt our ability to see the truth—the vagus nerve needs stimulation.

When we are sending mixed messages throughout our entire body, there are going to be many issues associated. All bodies react differently, so it's challenging to pinpoint the exact location symptoms are felt.

What you can do for yourself is to ensure that you are reflecting on your body. What is it that your body needs?

The best method of keeping track is to journal. You don't have to write a "Dear diary…" entry every day, but you should be keeping track of how you felt. Maybe it's simply a notes app on your phone, or you could track it more analytically in a spreadsheet.

Whatever you do, pay attention to how you felt throughout the day. You can go back and look at your week and think to yourself, "I'm anxious right before I go to work every day." You might notice you are the most relaxed when hanging out with a certain friend or participating in a specific activity.

This gives you the ability to know exactly what is required for your health. Give your body everything it needs to function optimally. Cut back on the things that stress you out or come up with healthy coping mechanisms. Be mindful of the things that provide you the most joy and put more of an effort toward nurturing these aspects.

The process of vagal stimulation is one where discussion is encouraged. Feel free to reach out with further questions and provide some feedback if you've managed to learn anything from this title!

Remember that this is an exciting journey that is going to result in greater health. You are making these choices for your body and nobody else's. You don't just need to stimulate the vagus nerve – you deserve to